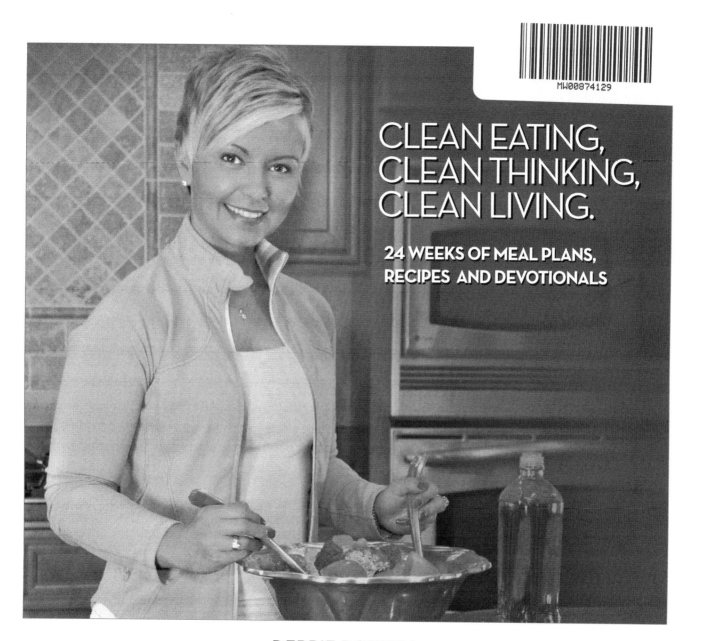

CLEAN EATING, CLEAN THINKING, CLEAN LIVING.

24 WEEKS OF MEAL PLANS, RECIPES AND DEVOTIONALS

DEBBIE PORTELL

CERTIFIED PERSONAL TRAINER AND NUTRITION COACH

WWW.DEBBIEPORTELL.COM

TABLE OF CONTENTS

INTRODUCTION

Eleven years ago I came home from a job in the financial industry where I constantly worked my little heart out. I sat at my dinner table with my usual fast food sandwich and fried potatoes. I drank it down with a usual soda and prepared my nightly drink, which was either a glass of wine or vodka martini. This night was different; I wasn't feeling well at all. I thought maybe I would feel better after my meal, but no such luck. I started to black out in my living room. Then I started to shake as if I was having convulsions. The ambulance came and rushed me to the hospital. My thyroid levels were a little off, but the doctors felt it was no reason for concern. My heart rate and blood pressure were elevated, but my blood count was low. I spent the next two years trying to figure out what happened to me that day and I didn't feel better, in fact I continued to feel worse. At one point I was 98 pounds. I couldn't eat anything without having a severe reaction. I would get dizzy, my heart rate would elevate, I would shake excessively, and I had migraines often.

Six months into this illness I had to quit my job that I loved so much and worked so hard to achieve. I couldn't make it through the day without thinking I needed to go to the ER. One day, I was home alone and I gave up. I gave up hope that I would ever get better. I was ready to die. To be put out of my misery. I laid in the bath tub and I cried out to just let it all come to an end. I went into my living room and turned on the TV, which I rarely watched. The first thing that came on was a man who said, "have you lost all hope? Do you feel like you will never get out of the situation you're in?" He said "there is hope in Jesus. Give your heart to the Lord today and pray this prayer with me and he will hear your cries." I fell to my knees and said the prayer out loud with that pastor on the TV. I didn't know what else to do. Where else could I turn? The doctors didn't know how to fix it.

After that day, my father brought me a Bible. He read it with me and prayed with me. I insisted I be baptized in case I didn't survive what I was going through. I read in the Bible, "If there is water what forbids you to be baptized?" It explained that this sacrament washes away the old you and allows the new creature that you have become in Christ to appear. I wanted to wash away the pain. The terrible illness that was riddling my body that *no* one could figure out.

So I did just that. I was baptized and I read that Bible day in and day out. The minute I got up, I had it in my hands and at night I would fall asleep with it on my chest. It was my way out of all of this darkness. There was hope in Jesus. I kept reading the promises of healing and I believed in my heart that God was able to heal me. He did heal me. It took me some time before I got the answers I needed in order to start feeling somewhat normal again, but I never lost faith that God would supply all of my needs just as his word said.

The turning point started when a friend recommended Dr. Christian Wessling to me. She said he helped her autistic son whom *no* one was able to help for years. She was right. The first thing he asked me was, "What is your blood type?" I had no idea. He tested me and the results showed I was type O. Boy was I eating wrong! I was previously sent to a registered dietician, so I was eating exactly what she suggested. I was eating various forms of dairy products and whole wheat foods, which she told me would help stabilize my blood sugar and prevent hypoglycemia. Turns out I was severely hypoglycemic, but it was reactive hypoglycemia, meaning everything I ate caused issues. As a blood type O, the two primary foods to avoid are wheat and dairy. I started feeling better within a day of changing my food. Keep in mind, I was sick for two years, quit my job, gave up on athletics, and was more or less dedicated to health.

With the help of Dr. Anna Bone, I was diagnosed with Hashimoto's Disease, an auto-immune disease of the thyroid. I started taking the medication Armour Thyroid and became very specific about my food. I must avoid wheat, dairy, corn, soy, coffee, chocolate, oats, peanuts and all forms of gluten.

I spent years studying health and nutrition. It was my life. In fact, my life depended on me finding an answer. I continued to seek the Lord for direction, so I could help others who might be in a similar situation. He opened the door and flooded me with opportunities and blessings I never imagined possible. I am a life changer. That is my position, title and function on this Earth. God aligns just the right people to find their way to me. Sometimes they are only there for a short time and others longer, but I instill as much as I can into each person.

Food serves two roles: a sustenance for life or a sentence to death. This is what I learned. I was killing myself with my food and I was under 30. I do have a disease that I will have until I die, but I am informed enough now to live the best life I can in spite of it. If I continued to eat the items on my list of "foods to avoid," I wouldn't be here to write this book. I would have a whole host of health issues, ultimately leading to a premature death.

My health is my most prized possession outside of my faith. I protect it like a strong warrior. No one will ever convince me to do otherwise. I go to bed at night when I should, I prepare my food weekly exactly as I should, I eat in the intervals needed so that I always feel my best. Nothing gets in the way of taking care of my health. If food is stealing your life, then switch gears, change channels or flip the switch. Come over to my side of the street. Live the best life you can today, each day. Food is food: it is not entertainment, it is survival. Food is not meant for short-term satisfaction, but for long-term gratification. Food is life or death. Choose life, eat clean!

What are these meal plans all about?

I started writing these meal plans a little over a year ago, shortly after my father had a heart attack. My dad is the strongest, smartest guy I know. He worked out six days a week my entire life. I have worked out with him for as long as I can remember. We swam together and played basketball, softball, golf and ice hockey (yes, that's right, even ice hockey) together. We lifted weights together since I was in the sixth grade. I couldn't believe it was really happening when they told me. It happened to him when he was at the gym with my mom. Unfortunately, she had to witness the event. She is one strong mama. They immediately "froze him," as we call it. His body temperature was dramatically lowered to prevent further organ damage. He was on a ventilator for two weeks because he had pneumonia. We couldn't fix the heart until we healed the pneumonia. I prayed Psalm 91 over him daily and the Lord delivered him from that. They were able to successfully perform a quadruple bypass and surgically insert a pacemaker.

2

My dad needed to make a serious change or he would go right back into a bad situation again. His exercise had helped him but his arteries were still blocked. His food had to be changed dramatically or he would be at risk for further complications. God spared my dad's life and plans to keep him around for many years to come. Not everyone can say that. I created Bill's Heart Healthy Menu because I started cooking my Dad's food for him from the first day he arrived home. Each week I prepare him an entire week's worth of food and on Sundays, we work together to separate it into daily portions. His health is great now. His lab values stay exactly the way they should and his weight stays exactly where it should. Before the heart attack, his weight didn't even out though his exercise was on track. His food needed adjusting. Food is life or death for you. Bill's Heart Healthy Menus are exactly what my dad eats each week. I hope that someone out there will be blessed by this information.

My menu is exactly what I eat each day to maintain my blood sugar. It also keeps me from having an auto-immune attack. Each of my menus is dairy, soy, corn and gluten free. I do not eat processed foods.

I eat out minimally, but when I do, I make my own sauces with lemon and olive oil. If I eat out I normally order a filet, steamed non-buttered veggies with lemon and olive oil on top or plain grilled chicken with a large salad without cheese, dressing or croutons. I add lemon and olive oil on top for my dressing.

The sample menu I create each week is for everyone else. It is a little more creative. It is mostly dairy-free, but I do add it in on some occasions. Just be aware. It is most certainly soy- and gluten-free. Everyone has a different metabolism. The best thing you can do is hire a professional that will sit down and evaluate your current nutrition; then, have them create a meal plan that is specific to you and your body's needs. When I meet with a new nutrition client I take into consideration the clients blood type, weight, height, health issues, medications, amount of hours awake, what time they fall asleep, how strenuous their occupation is, how much exercise they have within a day, their schedule and their likes and dislikes. If you meet with someone, please make sure they are addressing all of these items. Paying attention to everything you eat and drink for a full week will be

helpful information for them as well. It takes time; give everything about four weeks to take effect. If you cheat, plan five days before your body gets back on track, so you can plan to eliminate those five days from knowing how a plan is working. Cheating throws everything off, so don't beat yourself up, just know it will take time to reset all over again just as you did when you started.

Thank you for taking this journey with me. I pray that you are blessed by the experience.

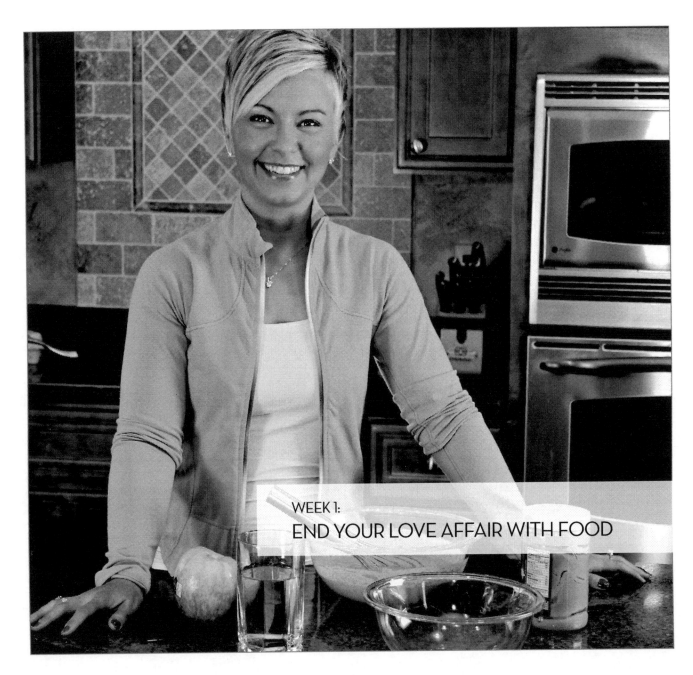

WEEK 1:
END YOUR LOVE AFFAIR WITH FOOD

All of you know my special health circumstances which require me to be very strict with my food. I don't see my views on health and nutrition as the only way or the only path to good health. There are many ways to achieve optimal health. This is simply the way I need to eat to support my immune system and my health. My purpose in presenting these meal plans to you each week is simply to motivate you to eat clean. To inspire you to make better choices. Most importantly, to help bring faith and peace into your day. My plans may or may not work for you for many reasons. These plans work for me because they are wheat-, soy-, dairy-, and corn-free. I am required to live without all of those due to my auto-immune disease. However, in my experience in working with clients on their nutrition, I have learned that so many folks have similar responses to these same foods. The best thing you can derive from my data is to understand that no two people are alike. You must find a way to learn how your body metabolizes food. Chicken simply might not be the right meat for you even though the American Heart Association says it

is. Take all the data you receive and hire a professional. Let them look at several things with you. First, your blood type. Some blood types have huge issues with certain foods and sometimes just avoiding those foods can change your life! Second, let them take a look at a year's worth of blood work. Each person has tendencies and a professional will be able to determine these tendencies. Third, keep a diary of what you eat and drink for a week and exactly how you feel after each meal. Maybe you are tired, weak, shaky, tachycardic, dizzy, moody, nauseous, constipated or whatever it is, keep track of it. This professional should be prepared to work with you for at least three months. It will take that long to test though a series of different foods. I suggest a book that my trainer suggested to me. It is "*How to Eat, Move and Be Healthy*" by Paul Chek. It has a detailed questionnaire which will help determine which macronutrient you process best: protein, carbohydrate, or fat.

This is only one aspect you should consider in your quest, but certainly a helpful one, just like the blood type.

THIS IS NOT AN OVERNIGHT PROCESS. THIS IS A LIFETIME JOURNEY AND MUST BE CHANGED EVERY STEP ALONG THE WAY AS LIFE CHANGES.

This is not an overnight process. This is a lifetime journey and must be changed every step along the way as life changes. We can't always do the exact same thing. I don't know many professionals that are skilled in nutrition in this detail, but the folks I do know are life changers. No one knows your body as much as you do, so you cannot expect a nutritionist to be a miracle worker, but they will go to battle with you and keep you on track. Usually the naysayers that complain about why a plan didn't work for them or why a professional couldn't help them are typically the folks that didn't put their heart into the program. They only gave it 80% but expected 100% results. You reap what you sow and having that type of mindset will not work in favor of your health.

After my dad recovered for a couple months, I thought to myself, "Wow I really need to get checked out for all of this." So I went out for a stress test, echocardiogram and very detailed blood work. Turns out everything is looking great for the heart. Thank the Lord! So I decided to do an experiment to see if I could improve at all. I decided for three months to eat only lean meats and significantly cut my fats and cholesterol. I ate only egg whites and chicken. Olive oil was my only fat source and I used it sparingly. I am an O blood type. My highly beneficial foods are beef, bison, salmon, olive oil, broccoli, and several others. I thought I would try to take the approach the dietician instructed my dad to follow, who is also blood type O. So I ate only chicken, turkey and egg whites for three months. When we went out, I only ordered chicken. The result of this three month experiment was that I experienced extreme fatigue, the exhaustion visible on my face and body. I barely made it through the day and was almost incapable of working out, despite my best efforts. I was sick three different times with a virus and had to go to the doctor for treatment

each time. No joke! My digestion was abnormal. My muscles felt achy daily, as if I had arthritis from head to toe. I experienced an acute migraine which was the first I had in my entire life and which lasted three days. I took two bottles of Ibuprofen total in three months and prior to that I had gone at least a year without taking it. I felt uncomfortably full and yet, hungry at the same time. At the end of the day around 7:30pm. I would fall asleep in my chair like a grandma. None of this is an exaggeration, it is exactly what happened to me. I went to my doctor again, and had my blood work repeated, and my numbers were worse. The total was higher in every area, The total values were higher in each area: fasting lipid panel, liver enzymes, vitamin D, vitamin B, liver enzymes, vitamin D, vitamin B, and renal functions were off.

Lesson Learned!
I am back on the plan!

Bison two times a day and salmon with dinner. My doctor looked at me on Thursday and said, "Debbie, what were you thinking? You know what

your body needs! Don't ever stop feeding your body what it needs." I took the time to type all of this to tell you that this is the real deal. Food is life or death for you. Make the choice to change your life and end your love affair with food. Roger always says, "It's only food," to his clients and he is right. Don't listen to the fad diets; always get a second opinion. The hospital dietitian suggested only lean meats and fat free foods for my dad. I serve him foods rich in fatty acids like salmon and olive oil. Within two days of changing my food, I felt normal again. Bison is loaded with B vitamins, necessary nutrients for me due to my auto-immune disease. Bison is high in niacin, a type of B vitamin that acts as a natural statin. It will lower your cholesterol! In some cases, chicken is higher in cholesterol than some cuts of bison. Before you change your food, think about what your eating and why.

Consider hiring a professional who really knows the ins and outs of nutrition to help you through the process. It is so much more than calories and carbs.
Trust me on this, you need to pay

attention to what you're putting in your body. Don't make me come to the hospital to have a nutrition session with you. Save your life and change your life now. It's not my way or the highway, remember that. I am just showing you the path I took and how it has impacted my life. My hope is that it will motivate you to make some changes. Something I believe in and feel everyone should consider is eating and buying organic. To be frank, it changed my life. My estrogen levels would have never changed if I had not moved to 18 organic eggs a day instead of 18 non-organic eggs a day. Everyone claims it is so expensive, but my Dad and I do it for our health. Maybe you might have to cut down on buying beer, cupcakes, Red Bulls, Diet Cokes or anything that does more harm than good to your health. Just try it for one month. Buy everything organic and tell me you don't feel better after a month. Next, read the book *"Eat Right for your Blood Type,"* by Peter Adamo. Please remember that this is not set in stone. If you are blood type A, I am not preparing you for a vegan lifestyle. However, I would like you to try to eliminate as many of the must-avoid foods as possible. Another thing I feel just as strongly about is not eating processed foods packed with preservatives. These preservatives are the exact reason why 13-year olds are walking around with a doughnut around their waistline and 30 year old men have declining testosterone levels. Processed foods are fake and full of chemicals that can be linked to all sorts of diseases I know you don't want. If you're going to eat eggs, crack the egg, don't eat, them out of a container. Or if you need a snack, don't grab for a bar with a paragraph of ingredients that appear to be in a foreign language. Finally, avoid artificial sweeteners. Aspartame is the devil. Read about it and actually understand what it is and what it does to your body. Attempt to use Stevia which is a plant, or agave which is a natural nectar. Better yet- learn to do without. These are the things I don't budge on. Yes you can continue to lose weight without following these rules, but I promise you a healthier life is ahead of you if you just try to follow these simple rules. Give it a month. Start today! Food, I am breaking up with you today! Our love affair has ended. My body is the temple of the Holy Spirit and from this point forward I will choose not to poison that with which God has so richly blessed me. Eat to live, do not live to eat. Trust me, when your health is gone, you will want it back and will wish you just took the time to make the change today.

"But those who hope in the Lord will renew their strength. They will soar on wings like eagles; they will run and not grow weary, they will walk and not be faint." Isaiah 40:31

Be an Eagle and soar your way through life. Have a wonderful week!

God Bless, Deb

SAMPLE MENU

BREAKFAST
2 omega egg omelet with chopped red, green and yellow peppers as well as onion. Topped with preservative-free and high fructose corn syrup-free organic salsa. Served with a cup of sliced strawberries

MID-MORNING SNACK
5 dried apricots dipped into 1 tbsp ground natural almond butter

LUNCH
5 oz Grilled Bison Sirloin Steak
1 cup spaghetti squash
1 cup roasted broccoli

MID-AFTERNOON SNACK
1 scoop vanilla Jay Robb egg white protein, with 1 tbsp ground natural almond butter blended with 1/2 tsp cinnamon.
1 pear

DINNER
5oz seasoned tilapia
1/2 cup mashed sweet potato
1 cup roasted broccoli

DEBBIE'S MENU

4 AM
Sweet Potato Pancake

7 AM
4 oz Bison Crock Pot Sirloin
2 cups baked green beans

10AM
Sweet Potato Pancake

1PM
4 oz Bison Chuck Roast
2 cups green beans

4PM
6 egg whites
2 cup steamed green beans with 1 tsp olive oil

7PM
5 oz Lemon Pepper Grilled Crunch Salmon
2 cups baked green beans

BILL'S HEART HEALTHY MENU

BREAKFAST
3 egg whites, scrambled
3/4 scoop chocolate Jay Robb egg white protein
1/2 banana

MID MORNING SNACK
1 Vanilla Apricot Protein Bar

LUNCH
5 oz Bison Mini-Meatloaf
1/4 cup brown rice
2 cups roasted broccoli
8 roasted carrots

AFTERNOON SNACK
2 containers applesauce
20 whole walnuts

DINNER
5 oz Lemon Garlic Tilapia
1/2 cup mashed sweet potato
1 1/2 cup mashed cauliflower

LEAD A HEALTHY, CLEAN LIFE BY CLEANSING YOUR BODY AND INSPIRING OTHERS WITH EVERYTHING YOU DO.

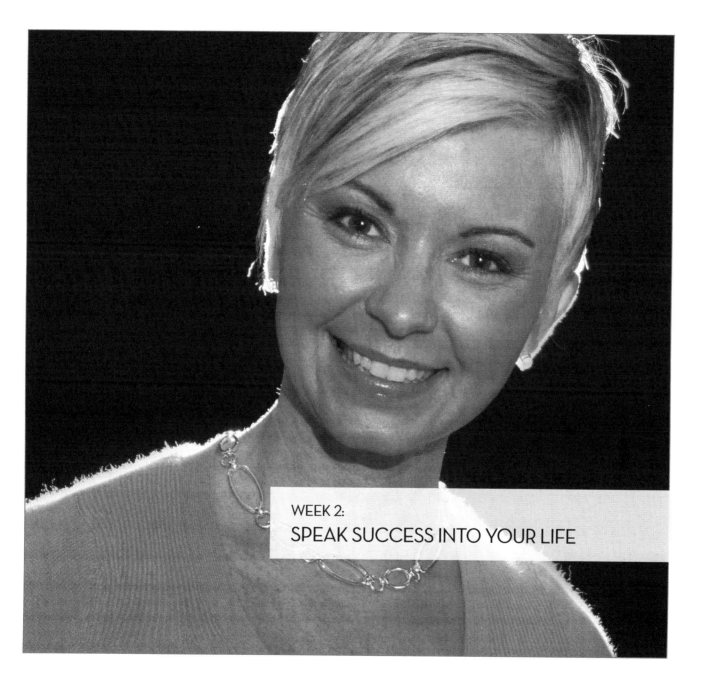

WEEK 2:
SPEAK SUCCESS INTO YOUR LIFE

How do you speak to yourself? What do you tell yourself you can or cannot do each day? Do you start each day with the motivation and drive to live life to its fullest, or do you start each day telling yourself what you can't do and all of the reasons why?

As a trainer and nutrition coach, I have met with folks who sabotage their success week after week just by the way they speak to themselves. When you look in the mirror, learn to love what you see. You may not be at your goal yet, but you are alive and God has given you the opportunity to live one more day.

Speak success into your life. Compliment yourself in your mind and never speak defeat out loud. Work hard and accept whatever level you're on, all the time knowing you will get further and further with hard work. However, more important than aesthetics is the fact that you're feeling better and better each day.

Remember: No excuses. A healthy life requires work, which includes time and dedication. Don't feel deflated and depressed about how hard it is to live healthy. Instead, feel blessed you have the ability to care for yourself and to continually improve your daily life.

My journey toward an all-around healthy lifestyle began ten years ago when I became bedridden and was uncertain each night when I fell asleep if I would have another day. Four months ago, when my father's heart stopped, we were thankful for each day he had in the hospital and praised God for each new day he gave us. Now, dad and I are healthier than ever! You may not have to experience a life-or-death situation to motivate you to better health, but don't wait until that. Live the best life you can now.

The bible says in 1st Corinthians 6:19, "Your body is a temple of the holy spirit." This reminds me each day that if my first priority is to live a life pleasing to God, then it matters what I put into my body. With my Hashimoto's Disease—the most common cause of hypothyroidism—I steer clear of obvious toxic behaviors such as alcohol and smoking, but food can be just as much of a poison to your body.

Represent the Lord through what he has given you with your body and how you choose to live. Remind yourself that you are a leader and an inspiration to others. Whether you know it or not, people are always watching you—especially the Father. So, lead a healthy, clean life by cleansing your body and inspiring others with everything you do. Make this the week that you change someone else's life just by living your own.

Make it a great week!

SAMPLE MENU

BREAKFAST
6 egg white cinnamon vanilla pancake
1/4 cup oatmeal
1 cup frozen blueberries with juice
on top of oats
2 tbsp peeled almonds,1 packet Stevia
and 1 tsp cinnamon on top of oats

MID-MORNING SNACK
No Bake Chocolate Cherry Protein bar

LUNCH
5 oz bake balsamic pineapple Salmon
2 cups steamed spinach with
3/4 cup balsamic onions recipe

MID-AFTERNOON SNACK
1 scoop vanilla Jay Robb egg white
protein powder 1/2 cup frozen
blueberries
1/2 cup frozen raspberries
1 tbsp barleans blueberry pomegranate flax oil blended in blender

DINNER
1 full bowl Chicken Chili

DESSERT
1 pear sautéed in an olive oil sprayed
skillet with 1 packet Stevia and
1 tsp cinnamon, cook on low heat
until cooked down and top with
1 tbsp almonds

DEBBIE'S MENU

4AM
6 egg whites
1 apple chopped mixed with 1
applesauce
2 tbsp almonds
1 packet Stevia and a dash of
cinnamon

7AM
5 oz Hulkburger
3.5 cups roasted squash

10AM
5 oz Hulkburger
3.5 cups roasted squash

1PM
5 oz Hulkburger
3.5 cups roasted squash

4PM
6 egg whites
1 pear chopped mixed with 1
applesauce
2 tbsp almonds
1 packet Stevia and a dash of
cinnamon

7PM
5 oz roasted turkey
3 cups green beans
2 tbsp apple cider vinegar onions
1 tbsp Agave chili sauce

BILL'S HEART HEALTHY MENU

BREAKFAST
3 egg whites, scrambled
1 scoop chocolate Jay Robb egg
white protein
1 banana
1 cup steel cut Irish oats

SNACK
1 Vanilla Apricot Protein Bar

LUNCH
5 oz Bison Mini Meatloaf
1 cup brown rice
2 cups Roasted Broccoli
8 Roasted Carrots

SNACK
2 containers applesauce
20 whole walnuts

DINNER
5 oz Roasted Turkey Breast
1 cup mashed sweet potato
1 1/2 cup mashed cauliflower

A HEALTHY LIFE REQUIRES WORK,
WHICH INCLUDES TIME AND
DEDICATION. DON'T FEEL DEFLATED
AND DEPRESSED ABOUT HOW HARD
IT IS TO LIVE HEALTHY.

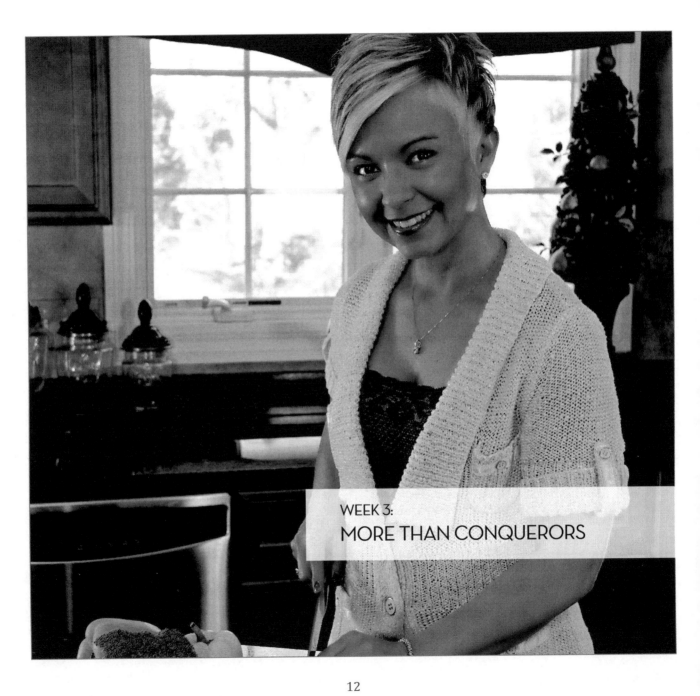

WEEK 3:
MORE THAN CONQUERORS

Learn to love your body and most importantly your life. Choose to look at each day as another opportunity instead of a hindrance. Lay down those feelings of heaviness. Try not to remember your failures and your difficulties, but instead choose to remember your victories. Life is only what you choose to make it.

Tell yourself each day you are a child of the most high God. You are walking in favor and blessings follow you in everything you do. Believe that your body can be healthy; believe that you have the strength and the courage to make the right decisions to be healthy everyday. Don't allow others to convince you to live differently.
As I've said before, do this first to please God, but do it for yourself and most importantly for your family. They need to see you lead! You are an inspiration to everyone you encounter!

Don't let anyone see you as anything other than the amazing person you are. No excuses! Just live the very best life you can, choose to do so every day and life will bless you.

In all these things, we are more than conquerors through him who loved us. Romans 8:37

TRY NOT TO REMEMBER YOUR FAILURES AND YOUR DIFFICULTIES,
BUT INSTEAD CHOOSE TO REMEMBER YOUR VICTORIES.
LIFE IS ONLY WHAT YOU CHOOSE TO MAKE IT.

SAMPLE MENU

BREAKFAST

1 whole egg, 4 egg whites whisked together with garlic pepper spice mix. Spray skillet and pour eggs on skillet. Finely chop 1 full cup Roasted Broccoli lay on top of eggs in skillet in the beginning, spread evenly, flip when cooked through. Top with picante sauce. Eat with 1 whole grapefruit with Stevia

MID-MORNING SNACK

No Bake apricot protein bar

LUNCH

Mustard Encrusted Tilapia
1 1/2 cup Roasted Broccoli
2 tbsp brown rice

MID-AFTERNOON SNACK

1 scoop chocolate Jay Robb egg white protein
1 tbsp chocolate raspberry flax oil
1 cup frozen raspberries all blended together.

DINNER

5 oz Roasted BBQ Chicken
12 spears roasted asparagus
1 bowl chow chow

DESSERT

1 pear sautéed in an olive oil sprayed skillet with 1 packet Stevia and 1 tsp cinnamon, cook on low heat until cooked down and top with 1 tbsp almonds

DEBBIE'S MENU

4AM

6 egg whites
1 pear chopped mixed with 1 applesauce
2 tbsp almonds
1 packet Stevia and a dash of cinnamon

7AM

1 scoop strawberry Jay Robb egg white protein powder
1 pear chopped mixed with 1 applesauce
2 tbsp almonds
1 packet Stevia and a dash of cinnamon

10AM

5 oz Shredded Bison
3 cups roasted squash

1PM

6 egg whites
1 pear chopped mixed with 1 applesauce
2 tbsp almonds
1 packet Stevia and a dash of cinnamon

4PM

1 scoop strawberry Jay Robb egg white protein powder
3.5 cups roasted zucchini

7PM

5 oz Shredded Bison
3 cups green beans
2 tbsp apple cider vinegar onions

BILL'S HEART HEALTHY MENU

BREAKFAST

3 egg whites, scrambled
1 scoop chocolate Jay Robb egg white protein
1 banana
1 cup steel cut Irish oats

SNACK

1 Vanilla Apricot Protein Bar

LUNCH

5 oz Bison Mini-Meatloaf
1 cup brown rice
2 cups Roasted Broccoli
8 Roasted Carrots

SNACK

2 containers applesauce,
20 whole walnuts

DINNER

5 oz Baked Tilapia
1/2 cup mashed sweet potato
1 1/2 cup mashed cauliflower

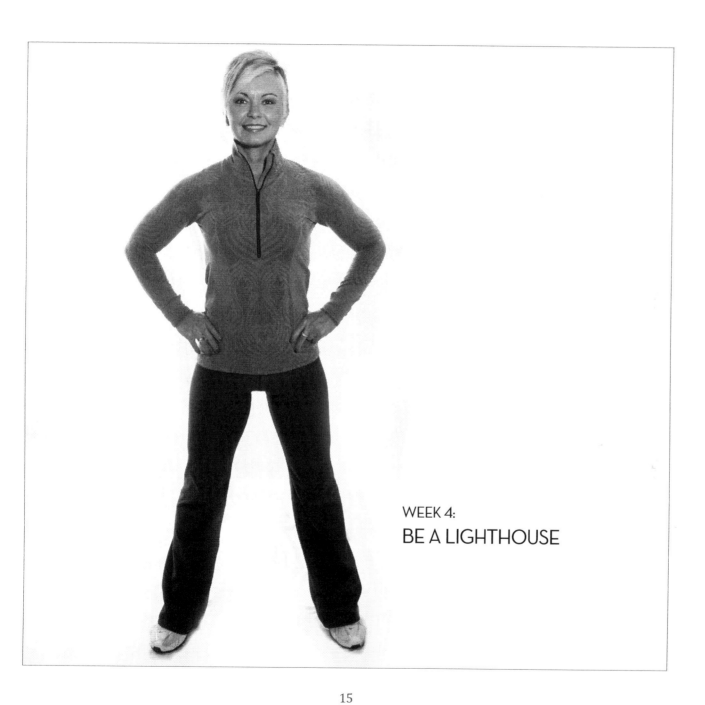

WEEK 4:
BE A LIGHTHOUSE

Do nothing out of selfish ambition or vain conceit, but in humility consider others better than yourselves. Each of you should look not only to your own interests, but also to the interests of others. Your attitude should be the same as that of Christ Jesus.
Philippians 2:3-5

I love this scripture because it reminds me daily to step out of my own world and realize there are much bigger things to consider. It is easy to let the daily hardships of life consume you. Family feuds, health issues, money issues, stress at work and just the basic obstacles in life can easily pile up on you in a day. Always remember you are blessed and not cursed! You are more than conquerors!

You are victorious!

We need to see our glass full even when the storms of life come. Even when things are piling up on our plate, we still have to muscle up and see the best in our day. Something can steal the joy in your life every day, but only if you allow it. Live in faith, live in expectancy of something great! Believe in favor and live life with a spirit of thankfulness. Don't focus on your obstacles; focus on your faith. Be humble and look outside yourself to see how you can please God and please others in everything you do.

I want to hold the Lueken family up in prayer. We lost a strong warrior this week, Mrs. Pat Lueken. Pat was a perfect example of all that I speak of each week. She trained in our gym twice a week and came in on her own daily. Exercise and fitness transformed her life during the time she spent at our gym. She was so blessed by her health improving. She would tell us each week how much better she was feeling. Rest in peace Pat Lueken. Your sweet smile and amazing spirit was an inspiration to all who encountered you. I feel blessed to have the opportunity I had to get to know Pat. We love the entire Lueken family and wish you the best. To be absent from the body is to be present with the Lord. She is a shining star who will shine her sweet spirit down on us each day.

Everyone keep pressing on! Life carries on each day and these struggles that we go through constitute our life. Don't let the storms of life stop you from showing your light. Be a lighthouse. Always be an inspiration to others. Watch how you speak, watch how you eat and drink, watch how you live in front of others. You don't realize who you are inspiring with your life. Make your life as bright as you can for others to see.

Pat, you made your life bright and you inspired me. God bless you and your family.

DON'T LET THE STORMS OF LIFE STOP YOU FROM SHOWING YOUR LIGHT. BE A LIGHTHOUSE. ALWAYS BE AN INSPIRATION TO OTHERS.

SAMPLE MENU

BREAKFAST

3 egg whites scrambled 3 oz ground
bison topped with 1/4 cup salsa
1/2 cup mixed berries mixed with
1 tbsp strawberry-banana flax oil

MID-MORNING SNACK

1 No Bake apricot protein bar

LUNCH

5 oz Tilapia Salad on top of a large
bed of mixed greens with 10 grape
tomatoes

MID-AFTERNOON SNACK

Cinnamon Vanilla Egg White Pancake
1 cup unsweetened applesauce
mixed with
15 walnuts

DINNER

5 oz Shredded BBQ Chicken
1 cup mashed sweet potato
1 cup roasted red pepper and onion

DEBBIE'S MENU

4AM

6 egg whites
1 pear chopped mixed with 1 applesauce
2 tbsp almonds
1 packet Stevia and a dash of cinnamon

7AM

5 oz Hulkburger
1 pear chopped mixed with 1 applesauce
2 tbsp almonds
1 packet Stevia and a dash of cinnamon

10AM

5 oz Shredded Bison
2 cups green beans

1PM

6 egg whites
2 cups Spaghetti Squash
1 tbsp Agave chili sauce

4PM

1 scoop strawberry Jay Robb egg
white protein powder
25 spears roasted asparagus

7PM

5 oz Shredded Bison
Large mixed green salad with tomatoes, onion, and cucumber mixed
with lemon vinaigrette

BILL'S HEART HEALTHY MENU

BREAKFAST

3 egg whites, scrambled
3/4 scoop chocolate Jay Robb egg
white protein
1/2 banana
1/4 cup steel cut Irish oats

SNACK

1 Cinnamon Roll Larabar

LUNCH

5 oz Bison Mini Meatloaf
1/4 cup brown rice
2 cups Roasted Broccoli
8 Roasted Carrots

SNACK

2 containers applesauce,
15 whole walnuts

DINNER

5 oz Agave Salmon
1/2 cup mashed sweet potato
1 1/2 cup Roasted Cauliflower

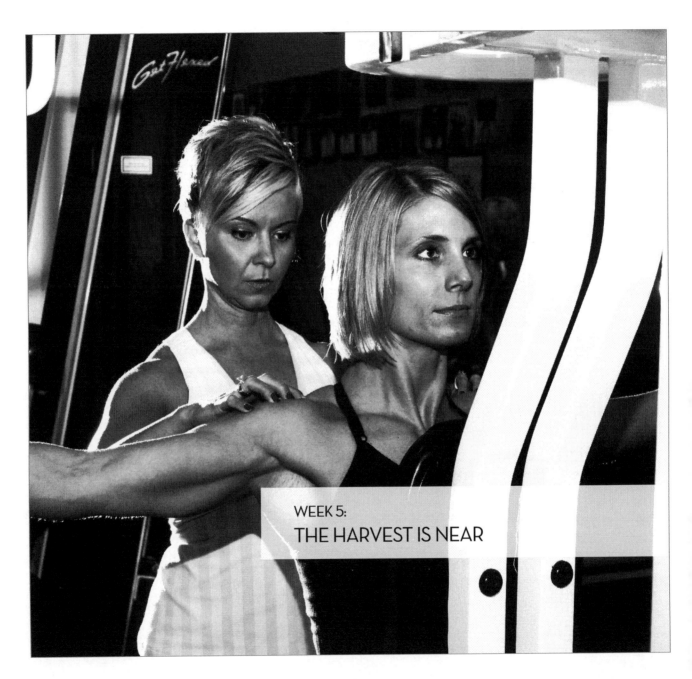

WEEK 5:

THE HARVEST IS NEAR

As a trainer and nutrition coach, I hear so many excuses for why folks have not continued with their programs. They come to me after many years of failures look at me and ask me why working with me is going to make things any different for them. I reply, "it won't be my doing, it will be your doing."

I'm simply a God-given tool to inject them with faith, confidence, determination, strength, favor and power. When they are weak, I will be strong for them. When they give up over and over and over again, I will never give up on them. When their world around them tells them to drink, smoke and binge, I will continue to live a life of example in front of them.

However, no matter how much I do, they are responsible for their destiny. I don't need posters of myself on the wall, videos of my achievements, or hallways filled with trophies to prove what I can do for them. It's not about me. It's about them.

Everyday in every aspect of life, we must choose not to grow weary in doing good, no matter the circumstances. Harvest is near! Favor is flowing! You are closer to your next blessing than you think. When life presents you with struggles, we cannot choose to turn to food, to wine, to drugs, to gossip or to whatever you are using to mask and block yourselves from living life to its fullest capacity.

We can wake up tomorrow and find out it's our last. When you really take inventory of your life each day, no matter the struggle ahead, you must choose to see the glass full.

So I say to that new client, "I won't make this change, you will. I am your trainer for life until you tell me I am not. Now let's get started changing your life." Whether it's weight loss, weight gain or health improvement, today is the day to flip the switch.

Choose health always. Live a better and fuller life because of it. When your heart is telling you not to eat something, drink something, smoke something or speak a defeated word, choose not to do so! Control your destiny. Don't grow weary doing good!

Don't quit! Harvest is near.

Have a great week.

SAMPLE MENU

BREAKFAST
1/3 cup oatmeal
1 cup mixed berries with
2 tbsp sliced almonds, mixed
together;
Cinnamon Vanilla Egg White Pancake

MID-MORNING SNACK
1 No Bake Strawberry Protein Bar

LUNCH
5 oz Melt in Your Mouth Roast
6 sweet potato fries
1 cup Roasted Broccoli with garlic

MID-AFTERNOON SNACK
1 scoop Jay Robb chocolate egg
white protein
1 tbsp chocolate raspberry flax oil
and 1 cup frozen raspberries
blended with water

DINNER
5 oz Agave grilled Salmon with
1/2 cup balsamic onions on top
1 plate full of grapefruit salad

AFTER DINNER SNACK
1 cup unsweetened applesauce with
12 walnuts on top mixed with
cinnamon and Stevia

DEBBIE'S MENU

4AM
6 egg whites
1 pear chopped mixed with 1 applesauce
2 tbsp almonds
1 packet Stevia and a dash of cinnamon

7AM
5 oz Hulkburger
2 cups Spaghetti Squash

10AM
5 oz Shredded Bison
2 cups Spaghetti Squash

1PM
1 scoop strawberry Jay Robb egg
white protein
1 tbsp strawberry banana flax oil
1 container applesauce

4PM
5 oz Shredded BBQ Chicken
2 cups Spaghetti Squash

7PM
5 oz Shredded Bison
2 cups green beans

BILL'S HEART HEALTHY MENU

BREAKFAST
3 egg whites, scrambled
3/4 scoop chocolate Jay Robb egg
white protein
1/2 banana
1/4 cup steel cut Irish oats

SNACK
1 Cinnamon Roll Larabar

LUNCH
5 oz Shredded BBQ Chicken
1/2 cup mashed sweet potato
1 1/2 cup Roasted Cauliflower

SNACK
2 containers applesauce
15 whole walnuts

DINNER
5 oz Bison Meatloaf
1/4 cup brown rice
2 cups Roasted Broccoli
8 Roasted Carrots

SO LET'S NOT ALLOW OURSELVES
TO GET FATIGUED DOING GOOD. AT
THE RIGHT TIME WE WILL HARVEST A
GOOD CROP IF WE DON'T GIVE UP,
OR QUIT. GALATIANS 6:9

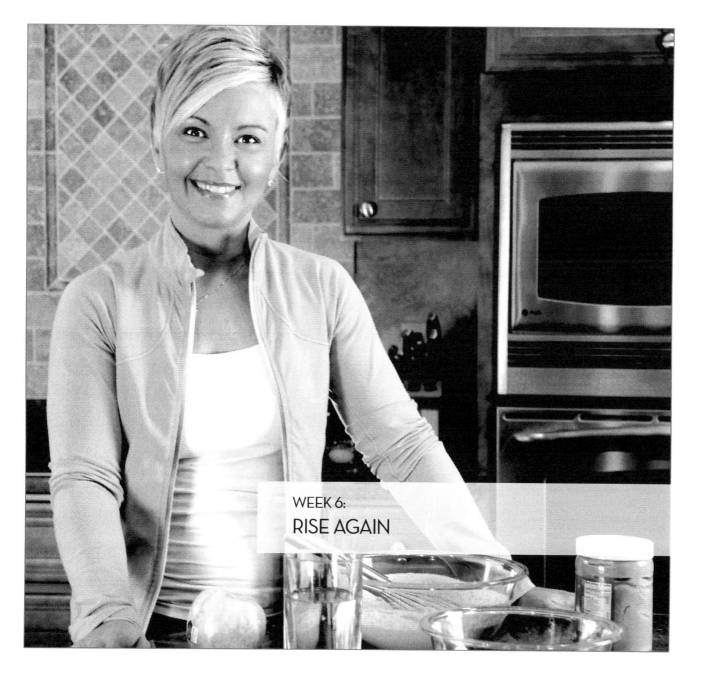

WEEK 6:
RISE AGAIN

For though a righteous man falls seven times, he rises again...
Proverbs 24:16

I like this scripture because it reminds me that it is OK to fail. Failure is a part of life. My largest failures have given rise to some of my most amazing accomplishments. I try so hard to learn from my mistakes and not repeat them, but life is not perfect and often times we can repeat our mistakes.

If you're struggling with your food or your exercise and it is causing health or self-esteem issues, rise again! It's time! Joel Osteen said, "Nobody can keep you from your destiny but you." Rise again. It is a new day. The past is the past. If yesterday's eating was terrible, then make today great. Don't get bitter, don't get negative and don't give up! Rise again! It is never too late to start fresh and make a new life for yourself. You haven't made too many mistakes, you aren't too old, you're not too busy, you're not a failure. Rise again!

Each day is a new day for a fresh start. Start it up! Today is the day! Eat clean, do your cardio, get your workout in, read a passage, compliment someone, or tell your spouse they are beautiful and you love them. Start a new day today.

Joel also said, "This is a new day.... It may not have happened in the past, but it will happen someday." I know God has favor coming my way. Declare that for yourself every day. Your time is coming. Stay in faith and clear out the negative clutter in your mind. Replace it with thoughts of praise, joy and peace. I'M SERIOUS! Do it! Instead of saying, "I am so tired, I haven't slept all night," say, "Today is going to be a great day." Instead of saying, "I ate so bad this week, I feel awful and I don't fit into anything," say, "I am a child of the most high God, I am blessed and not cursed, I am going to eat great today and feel wonderful and look wonderful because of it."

Find a way to tap into good energy. Everyone has lived in a world surrounded by negative energy before. Don't let them steal your joy. Fight! Fight 'til the death! Go to the mattresses! Don't let them get inside you. Try buying a daily devotional calendar, post quotes on your wall, pray and praise God for his goodness. On my lunch break, I check out the website for my church - St. Louis Family Church - in Chesterfield, slfc. com. My pastor has great podcasts. Wow, I feel charged up after these! If this is not your taste, then do what it takes to make yourself happy. Don't speak negative thoughts to yourself. Those thoughts are toxic and introduce disease to your body and to the lives of others surrounding you.

Let your light shine in everything you do! Be an inspiration starting today. You can do this. Don't you dare tell yourself you can't.

God Bless.

SAMPLE MENU

BREAKFAST
Pumpkin Pancake
1 cup berries
1 tbsp almond butter with Stevia and
cinnamon- spread on top of pancake

MID-MORNING SNACK
1 No Bake Apricot protein bar

LUNCH
5 oz Ezekiel Bread Encrusted
Chicken Cutlet
1 cup Spaghetti Squash with
1 tbsp chili sauce
1 cup steamed green beans with
garlic pepper seasoning

MID-AFTERNOON SNACK
1 scoop vanilla Jay Robb protein
1 tbsp cinnamon Stevia almond butter
1/2 banana

DINNER
5 oz French Onion Bison Beef Tips
on top of
1 cup Spelt Pasta noodles
Salad on side with red pepper, red onion,
pepperoncini, olive oil, balsamic
vinegar, garlic pepper, onion powder
whisked together
12 walnuts on top mixed with
cinnamon and Stevia

DEBBIE'S MENU

4AM
6 egg whites
1 pear chopped mixed with 1 applesauce
2 tbsp almonds
1 packet Stevia and a dash of cinnamon

7AM
5 oz Hulkburger
2 cups Spaghetti Squash

10AM
5 oz Hulkburger
2 cups Spaghetti Squash

1PM
5 oz Hulkburger
2 cups Spaghetti Squash

4PM
6 egg whites
1 scoop Clear-Vite
1 tbsp chocolate raspberry flax oil
1 container applesauce

7PM
5 oz Grain-Free Turkey Meatloaf
2 cups green beans

BILL'S HEART HEALTHY MENU

BREAKFAST
3 egg whites, scrambled
3/4 scoop chocolate Jay Robb egg
white protein
1/2 banana
1/4 cup steel cut Irish oats

SNACK
1 Cinnamon Roll Larabar

LUNCH
5 oz Bison Mini Meatloaf
1/4 cup brown rice
2 cups Roasted Broccoli
8 Roasted Carrots

SNACK
2 containers applesauce
15 whole walnuts

DINNER
5 oz Lemon Tilapia or Agave Salmon
1/4 cup brown rice
2 cups Roasted Broccoli
8 Roasted Carrots

RISE AGAIN. IT IS A NEW DAY.
THE PAST IS THE PAST.
IF YESTERDAY'S EATING WAS TERRIBLE,
THEN MAKE TODAY GREAT.

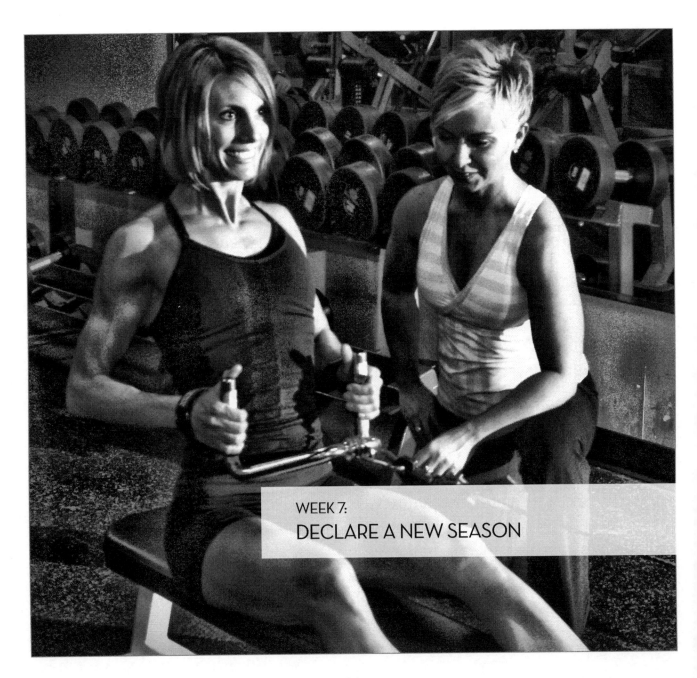

WEEK 7:
DECLARE A NEW SEASON

"What the enemy intends for your harm, God will turn around and use to your advantage." John 10:10

Another version of this scripture says, "The thief comes only to steal and kill and destroy, I have come that they may have life and have it to the full." I love this version. Who is your thief? Who is trying to steal, kill and destroy your dreams, your joy, your peace? It may not be someone else, it may be yourself. Your own negative thoughts can rob your life of progress.

Declare a new season for your life, just like a coach must do for a losing football team. He must press forward toward the goal of winning the next season. He cannot remain in the past or his team will lose again. Joel Osteen said, "Every setback is simply a setup for a comeback." Set it up! Let's come back strong. Tomorrow is the best day to start. Eat clean, do your cardio, get into the gym, speak positive words to yourself and to your family. It doesn't matter what you did wrong yesterday.

That is the past. It is time to change the present. Don't let the thief convince you that you are too busy or that you're not good enough.

We all have obstacles to overcome. Mine is a daily battle with my health. My food is how I survive. I can see this as a setback or I can see it as what sets me aside from the rest! No matter what challenge I have encountered in my life (and there are plenty), I speak faith that I will overcome the challenge and great blessings will come my way.

Choose to keep your distance from toxins. This not only includes processed foods, sugars, alcohol, and smoking, but even more importantly, friends and family that dump their trash of negative energy on you. Don't gossip with them or you will become toxic too. Keep your distance from folks who only feed you negative energy, walk in love, spread your joy to all and try to inspire them to be better simply by living a better life in front of them. Just don't let them in. Similar to the coach, if he has a player

that continually misses practice and doesn't give his all at the games, he would either have to work to rebuild that player or let them go. Otherwise that player will bring the team down.

I ask you today, "Who is your thief?" Your friends forcing you to drink and live a lifestyle you don't belong in because you are trying to choose health? Your job, your family, your thoughts or is it your excuses? God came so we could have life and live it to the fullest possible. Only connect with folks that make your team more successful. Eat clean! Do your cardio! Prepare your food!

SAMPLE MENU

BREAKFAST

2 whole eggs scrambled and topped
with 1/4 cup salsa
1 apple and 1 pear sautéed and
topped with Stevia and cinnamon

MID-MORNING SNACK

1 No Bake Chocolate Cherry
Protein Bar

LUNCH

5 oz Baked Balsamic Pineapple
Salmon
18 spears Balsamic Asparagus with
1 cup crushed pineapple (no syrup,
juice only)

MID-AFTERNOON SNACK

1 scoop strawberry Jay Robb egg
white protein powder
1 tbsp strawberry banana flax oil
6 frozen strawberries blended
with water

DINNER

5 oz Spicy Pan-Seared Chicken
2 cups Roasted Broccoli with garlic
and
1 cup Roasted Cauliflower

DEBBIE'S MENU

5AM

6 organic egg whites into an omelet
1 cup baked green beans
8 strawberries

8AM

4 oz Bison Crock Pot Sirloin Steak
with Schultz Hot Sauce on top
1 cup Spaghetti Squash
1 cup steamed green beans

11AM

5 oz Grilled Chicken Breast with
Debbie's Seasoning
and Schultz Hot Sauce on top
1 cup Spaghetti Squash
1 cup steamed green beans

2PM

6 egg white omelet
1 cup baked green beans
1 cup Spaghetti Squash
8 strawberries

5PM

5 oz Grilled Chicken Breast with
Debbie's Seasoning
and Schultz Hot Sauce on Top
2 1/2 cup Spaghetti Squash
1/2 cup sautéed leeks

BILL'S HEART HEALTHY MENU

BREAKFAST

3 egg whites, scrambled
3/4 scoop chocolate Jay Robb egg
white protein
1/2 banana
1/4 cup steel cut Irish oats

SNACK

1 Cinnamon Roll Larabar

LUNCH

5 oz Bison Mini Meatloaf
1/4 cup brown rice
2 cups Roasted Broccoli
8 Roasted Carrots

SNACK

2 containers applesauce
15 whole walnuts

DINNER

5 oz Lemon Tilapia or Agave Salmon
1/4 cup brown rice
2 cups Roasted Broccoli
8 Roasted Carrots

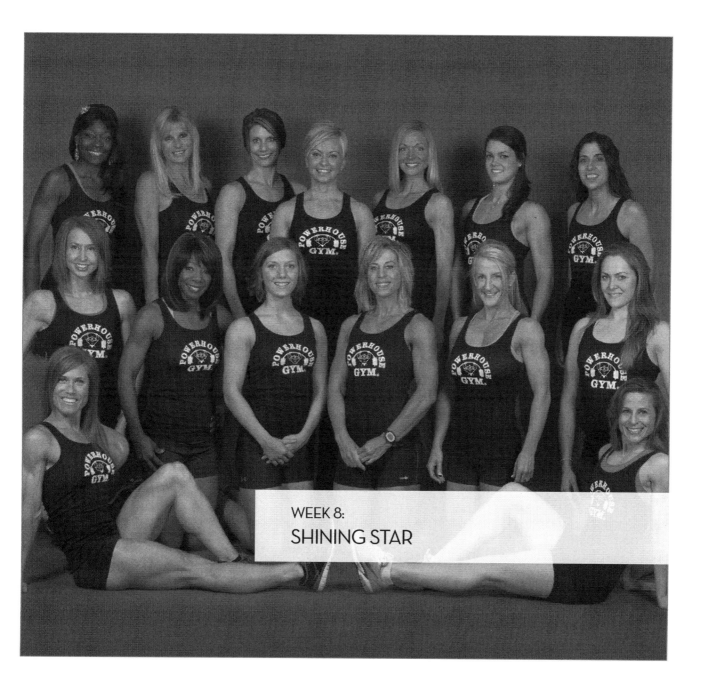

WEEK 8:
SHINING STAR

27

*Do everything without grumbling
or arguing, so that you may become
blameless and pure "children of God"
without fault in a warped and crooked
generation. Then you will shine like
stars in the sky as you hold firmly to
the word of life.
Philippians 2:14-16*

Do you stand out for being different, for being positive? Joel Osteen said, "Life is too short to hang around negative, critical, judgmental and jealous people...Get around people who will stir up seeds of greatness in you." Find some dreamers! People who build you up!

I have two points to this message. Who is holding you back? Who is keeping your star from shining? Who promotes you to become negative? Who pressures you to drink when you know you shouldn't, to eat when you know you shouldn't or simply to grumble and wallow in negative energy together? Don't let anyone do this to you. Don't let anyone tell you "no" or that you cannot do something. Don't let anyone keep you from your dreams. If your dream is to live a healthy and fit lifestyle, then don't let anyone, and I mean anyone tell you that you can't. Be a shining star. Shine so brightly that even the most negative people cannot penetrate your joy. Be contagious. Don't provide a toxic person an environment to flourish. Negative people will suffocate if you continually bless them with kindness and peace.

Lastly, if you are holding yourself back, then stop. Today is a good day to start. Get to the gym, get your cardio and workout in. You don't need anyone's approval, just get there and do it. Choose clean food and choose not to overindulge. Food is not a hobby, nor an activity. It is simply what our body requires to survive. I work hard each week to create new ways to prepare healthy food that work within the parameters of a healthy framework for most folks. Choose health. Food is not your hobby. Prepare your food for the week and be thankful that you are able to do so.

Do everything without grumbling or arguing, so that you may become blameless and pure "children of God". Be a shining star folks. Love the life you live. Clear out the limitations you have placed on yourself and live a limitless life. Don't let your friends, coworkers or family convince or influence you to live differently. Think about increasing! Increase health and defeat the limited, "I can't do it, it's too hard, I'm too busy, I have kids, I have failed too much" mentality and turn it into victorious, "I can do all things through Christ who strengthens me" mentality!

Shift your thoughts of lack to favor and never let any negative person steal your joy in life, but always pray for them. Control your destiny by controlling your thoughts.

SAMPLE MENU

BREAKFAST
Cinnamon Vanilla Egg White Pancake
1/2 cup frozen peaches mixed with
2 tbsp almonds

MID-MORNING SNACK
1 Cinnamon Roll Larabar

LUNCH
5 oz tilapia salad
12 spears roasted asparagus
1 cup mixed berries

MID-AFTERNOON SNACK
1 scoop vanilla Jay Robb egg white
protein blended with
1 tbsp almond butter and
1/4 cup oatmeal

DINNER
5 oz Roasted BBQ Chicken
2 cups Chow Chow
1 cup frozen spinach steamed with
apple cider vinegar, olive oil, garlic
powder, and pepper

DEBBIE'S MENU

4AM
6 egg whites
1 pear chopped mixed with 1 container applesauce
2 tbsp almonds
1 packet Stevia and a dash of cinnamon

7AM
5 oz Hulkburger
2 cups Spaghetti Squash
1 cup green beans

10AM
5 oz Hulkburger
2 cups Spaghetti Squash
1 cup green beans

1PM
5 oz Tilapia with 1 tbsp chili sauce
2 cups Spaghetti Squash
1 cup green beans

4PM
6 egg whites
1 apple chopped mixed with
1 container applesauce
2 tbsp almonds

7PM
5 oz Grain-Free Turkey Meatloaf
2 cups cucumber and 1 cup cherry
tomatoes mixed with olive oil, lemon
juice, apple cider vinegar, and Stevia

BILL'S HEART HEALTHY MENU

BREAKFAST
3 egg whites, scrambled
3/4 scoop chocolate Jay Robb egg
white protein
1/2 banana
1/4 cup steel cut Irish oats

SNACK
1 Cinnamon Roll Larabar

LUNCH
5 oz Bison Mini Meatloaf or 5 oz
Agave Salmon
1/2 cup mashed sweet potato
2 cups Roasted Broccoli
8 Roasted Carrots

SNACK
2 containers applesauce
15 whole walnuts

DINNER
5 oz Turkey Meatloaf
1/4 cup brown rice
2 cups Roasted Cauliflower

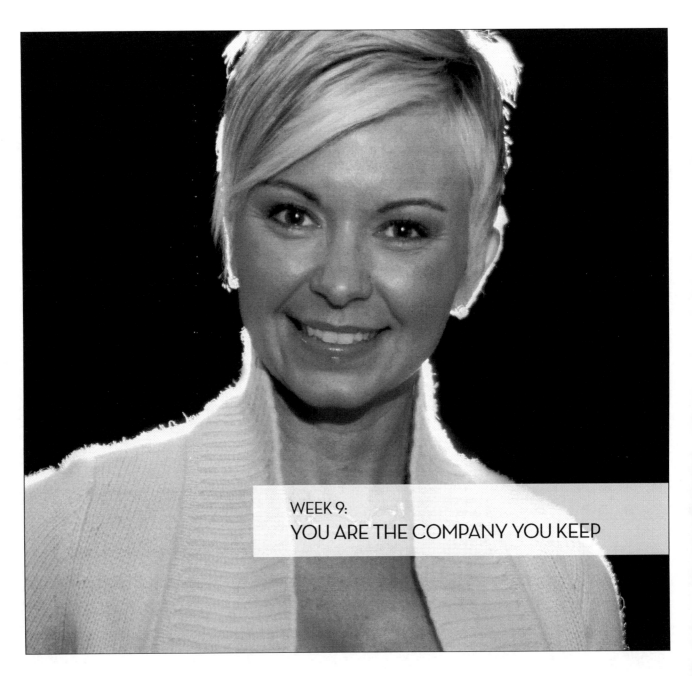

WEEK 9:
YOU ARE THE COMPANY YOU KEEP

I know what it is to be in need, and I know what it is to have plenty. I have learned the secret of being content in any and every situation, whether well fed or hungry, whether living in plenty or in want. Philippians 4:12

I once had a boss years ago tell me, "You are the company you keep, Debbie. If you choose to have lunch with the less aggressive, first to leave and last to arrive crowd, then you are likely to end up just like them." I ate lunch at my desk after that. Over the years, I have realized this couldn't be more true. If you build a foundation of people who support your dreams, your habits, your goals and your health aspirations, you are likely to be and remain successful in all areas of your life. If you surround yourself around negative, jealous, unhealthy people who don't understand why you work so hard for your health, then I guarantee you will fight tooth and nail to lose every pound.

My boss wanted me to stand out; she saw something in me and believed in me. I spent my time around her and other successful people. At a young age, I tried to model myself like them in hopes to achieve the same success. I wore a suit every day, came in 30 minutes early and stayed 30 minutes late. It worked. I surrounded myself with successful people and success came.

When it comes to a healthy lifestyle, you will find pitfalls around every corner. Several reasons to quit, to cheat, or to give into your friends or family so you don't stand out. Unearth a spirit of success inside you. Defeat is not an option. Your energy will be contagious to all of those around you and they too will want to make the same changes.

If your friends and family don't understand why you need to do your cardio daily, why Saturday afternoon you need to prepare your food for the week, why you cannot overeat and binge drink, don't let it get you down. You are not alone and never will be. First and foremost, you have me, and I will never give up on you and your success. We will fight to the death for it! Second of all, you have faith in knowing your body is a temple of the Holy Spirit and the more you live a life pleasing to God, the more blessings and favor will come your way. Finally, your health is your most important asset. Guard it with your life because having it is even more important than fitting into those skinny jeans.

No excuses this week. Clean eating, consistent cardio, and strength training equal optimal health which will bring you closer to living a life of which you have always dreamed. God bless you this week! Be strong, resist temptation, and inspire others with your passion and drive.

You can do this! Have a great week.
Deb

SAMPLE MENU

BREAKFAST
1 Pumpkin Pancake with
1 tbsp almond butter,
cinnamon and Stevia on top
1 cup sliced strawberries

MID-MORNING SNACK
1 No Bake Apricot Protein Bar

LUNCH
5 oz Cranberry Pineapple Salmon
on top of
2 cups spinach drizzled with
1/2 tbsp olive oil

MID-AFTERNOON SNACK
1 scoop vanilla Jay Robb egg white
protein blended with
1 cup frozen blueberries and
1 tbsp Barlean's blueberry
pomegranate flax oil

DINNER
5 oz Hot Chicken Salad
6 slices of tomato with 1 tbsp balsamic vinegar and
1 tsp olive oil
1 cup kale chips

DEBBIE'S MENU

4AM
6 egg whites
1 cup green beans
1/2 cup mashed sweet potato with
2 tbsp almonds

7AM
5 oz shredded BBQ chicken
2 cups Spaghetti Squash with
1 cup green beans, 1 tsp olive oil

10AM
5 oz BBQ Shredded Chicken
1 cup green beans
1/2 cup mashed sweet potato with
2 tbsp almonds

1PM
5 oz Pan-Seared Chicken
2 cups Spaghetti Squash with 1 cup
green beans and 1 tsp olive oil

4PM
6 egg whites
2 cups Spaghetti Squash
1/2 cup sweet potato, 1 tsp olive oil

7PM
1 scoop strawberry Jay Robb egg
white protein
2 cups Roasted Broccoli
1 cup Spaghetti Squash with 1 tsp
olive oil

BILL'S HEART HEALTHY MENU

BREAKFAST
3 egg whites, scrambled
3/4 scoop chocolate Jay Robb egg
white protein
1/2 banana
1/4 cup steel cut Irish oats

SNACK
1 Cinnamon Roll Larabar

LUNCH
5 oz Pan-Seared Chicken
1/2 cup mashed sweet potato
2 cups Roasted Cauliflower

SNACK
2 containers applesauce
15 whole walnuts

DINNER
5 oz BBQ Shredded Bison
1 cup Roasted Broccoli
2 tbsp brown rice
8 Roasted Carrots

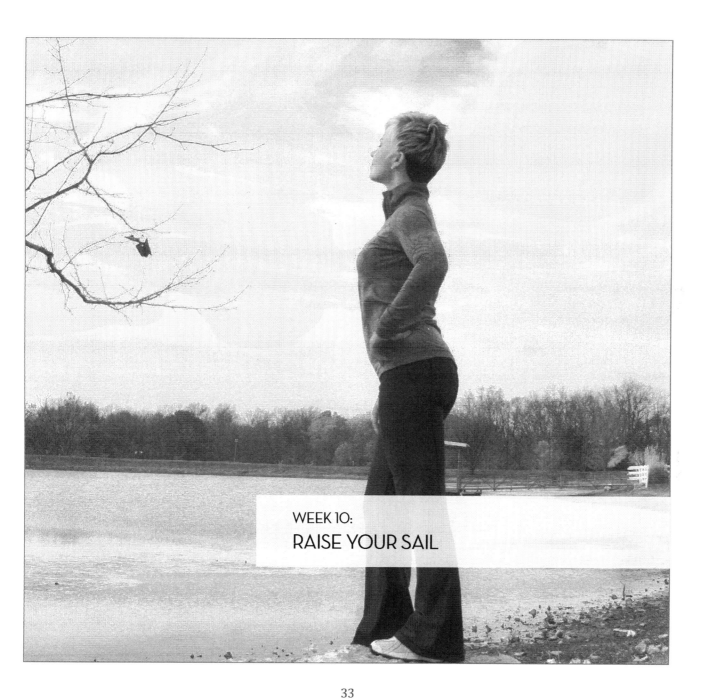

WEEK 10:
RAISE YOUR SAIL

Finally, brothers and sisters, whatever is true, whatever is noble, whatever is right, whatever is pure, whatever is lovely, whatever is admirable - if anything is excellent or praiseworthy - think about such things.
Philippians 4:8

Joel Osteen says, "God wants this to be the best time of your life. But, if you are going to receive this favor, you must enlarge your vision." You can't go around thinking negative, defeated, limiting thoughts and expect change or blessing.

Start each day out right. Today my pastor said to start your day by raising your sails. Put aside some time each morning to clear your mind of all negative energy. Press the reset button and clear your mind. Tune into what God has in store for you, your day and your life.

Get a vision in your mind of the life you want to live, the health you want to have, the body you want to achieve, and the world you want to live in. Speak words of faith and have thoughts of victory toward these goals. Stop the limited thinking and thoughts of defeat.

This week will be a great week for each of you. Build a strong foundation of success with your own thoughts; shift from thoughts of lack to thoughts of abundance. Tap into the people in your life who have good energy. Don't say you don't have anyone, because you have me and I am not going anywhere. Surround yourself around folks who care about their bodies and respect what they put in them. If overindulging in food and alcohol is not your thing, especially if it is making you sick and overweight, then quit! Don't let others lead you down a path of failure. You are not a failure; you are a winner. You are victorious.

You can do this. Make this a great week. Prepare your food! Do your cardio! Get your stretching and foam rolling in every day! Read words of success on a daily basis. Buy a devotional book or one that represents something positive to you. I like Joel Osteen and the Bible, but read what you love. Start your day with a few pages of that and watch the energy grow throughout your day. Compliment everyone you can, walk in love with everyone you encounter and most importantly, be happy with yourself and all that you have accomplished.

Keep pressing on, Deb

SAMPLE MENU

BREAKFAST
1 scoop chocolate Jay Robb egg
white protein powder
1 cup organic plain yogurt
1 cup frozen raspberries
1/4 cup steel cut oats – blended all
together

MID-MORNING SNACK
1 Cherry Pie Larabar

LUNCH
5 oz Bison Roast
6 baked sweet potato fries
10 spears roasted Balsamic Asparagus

MID-AFTERNOON SNACK
Cinnamon Vanilla Egg White Pancake
1 apple dipped into
1 tbsp almond butter

DINNER
5 oz chicken fingers
A large salad with celery, onion, and
red pepper with
1 tbsp apple cider vinegar
1 tsp olive oil, and
1 slice squeezed lemon

DEBBIE'S MENU

4AM
1 scoop strawberry Jay Robb egg
white protein
1 cup green beans
1/2 cup mashed sweet potato with
2 tbsp almonds

7AM
5 oz Pan-Seared Chicken
2 cups Spaghetti Squash
1 cup green beans
1 tsp olive oil

10AM
6.5 oz Grain-Free Turkey Meatloaf
1 cup green beans
1/2 cup mashed sweet potato

1PM
5 oz Pan-Seared Chicken
2 cups Spaghetti Squash
1 cup green beans with 1 tsp olive oil

4PM
1 scoop strawberry Jay Robb egg
white protein
1 cup green beans
1/2 cup mashed sweet potato

7PM
6.5 oz Grain-Free Turkey Meatloaf
2 cups Spaghetti Squash
1 cup green beans

BILL'S HEART HEALTHY MENU

BREAKFAST
3 egg whites, scrambled
3/4 scoop chocolate Jay Robb egg
white protein
1/2 banana
1/4 cup steel cut Irish oats

SNACK
1 Cinnamon Roll Larabar

LUNCH
7 oz Agave Salmon
2 cups Roasted Broccoli
8 Roasted Carrots

SNACK
2 containers applesauce
15 whole walnuts

DINNER
5 oz Turkey Meatloaf
1/2 cup mashed sweet potato
1 cup mashed cauliflower

STOP THE LIMITED THINKING AND
THOUGHTS OF DEFEAT.

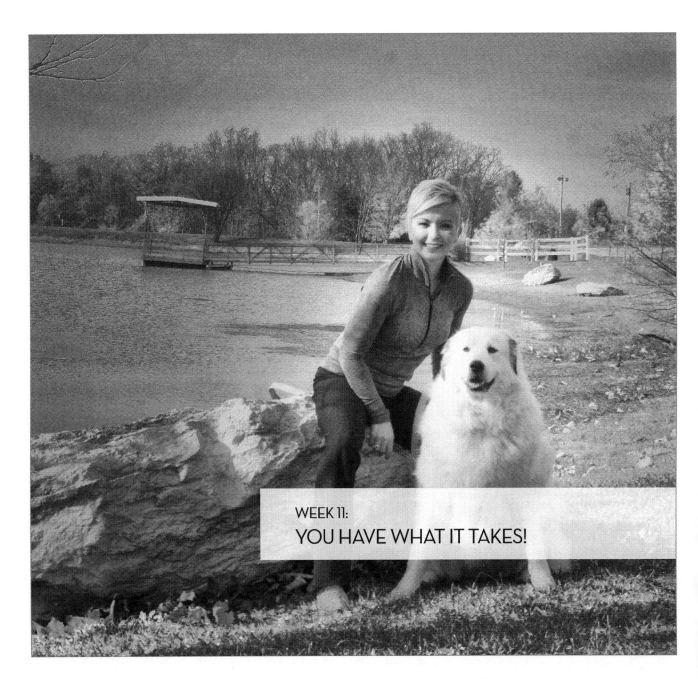

WEEK 11:
YOU HAVE WHAT IT TAKES!

"With long life I will satisfy him and show him my salvation" Psalm 91:16.

Don't make the mistake of always feeling bad about yourself. God knows you are not perfect and that you are going to make mistakes. Start believing that you have what it takes.

You have what it takes to be successful. What does that mean for you? Weight loss, financial stability, improved relationships or a better self-image? You have what it takes to achieve this.

When my father was in the hospital for 41 days, I would declare Psalm 91 over him daily. I would take each verse and receive it for him. I would digest the meaning of the verse as if it were my last meal. The last line says, "With long life I will satisfy you." It clicked after the first day that I wouldn't pray for my dad merely to survive; I prayed for a rapid recovery and declared long life over him. God said with long life he will satisfy you. You have what it takes. You are well equipped.

Past mistakes are in the past. Today is the day to change. I have recently gone through thorough testing to ensure my cardiovascular health is up to par, since I have an apparent genetic predisposition to cardiovascular disease. My cholesterol is a total of 135. My blood pressure is 105/60 with a heart rate of 68. I actually have to make sure I don't consume too much fish and magnesium or my blood pressure will go too low. Your health can change dramatically today just by changing what you put in your body. Simply eat clean on a regular basis and choose foods that promote health and demote disease.

Everything I put in my body has a purpose and positive benefit. My oils extend my cardiovascular health. My vegetables and fruits have specific vitamins and minerals that keep my energy levels where they need to be and help me to fight disease. The organic meats I eat are prepared fresh and provide my muscles the fuel they need to protect my bones and burn fat naturally.

I am giving you a foundation with these food plans. I recommend meeting with Roger or myself for a personalized plan, but clearly you know how to get started on a path of optimal health. Each week I send you several options.

Read Psalm 91. It's powerful stuff. Prepare your food this week, do your cardio and get to the gym and do your workouts. Listen, you've got what it takes! With long life God will satisfy you. Believe it and receive it for your life today. Make a decision today to make every minute count.

God bless and have a great week!

SAMPLE MENU

BREAKFAST
1 scoop chocolate Jay Robb egg white protein with
1 cup unsweetened almond milk
1/2 cup oats with 1 tbsp chocolate flax oil

MID-MORNING SNACK
2 organic mozzarella sticks
8 strawberries

LUNCH
5 oz Bison Meatloaf
2 cups baked green beans
1 cup frozen peaches (defrosted)

MID-AFTERNOON SNACK
25 almonds
8 strawberries

DINNER
5 oz Chicken Wingettes
2 cups Lemon-Pepper Roasted Broccoli

PRE-BEDTIME SNACK
1 cup unsweetened almond milk
1/2 scoop chocolate Jay Robb egg white protein

DEBBIE'S MENU

4AM
1 scoop strawberry Jay Robb egg white protein
1 cup green beans
1/2 cup mashed sweet potato with
2 tbsp almonds

7AM
5 oz shredded BBQ Chicken
2 cups baked green beans

10AM
5 oz Pan-Seared Chicken
12 spears roasted asparagus
1/2 cup mashed sweet potato

1PM
6 egg white pancake
2 cups baked green beans

4PM
6 egg white pancake
12 spears roasted asparagus
1/2 cup mashed sweet potato

7PM
5 oz Pan-Seared Chicken
3 cups Roasted Broccoli

BILL'S HEART HEALTHY MENU

BREAKFAST
3 egg whites, scrambled
3/4 scoop chocolate Jay Robb egg white protein
1/2 banana
1/4 cup steel cut Irish oats

SNACK
1 Cinnamon Roll Larabar

LUNCH
5 oz Shredded BBQ Chicken
1/2 cup mashed sweet potato
1 1/2 cup mashed cauliflower

SNACK
2 containers applesauce
15 whole walnuts

DINNER
5 oz Agave Salmon
2 cups Roasted Broccoli
8 Roasted Carrots
2 tbsp brown rice

PAST MISTAKES ARE IN THE PAST.
TODAY IS THE DAY TO CHANGE

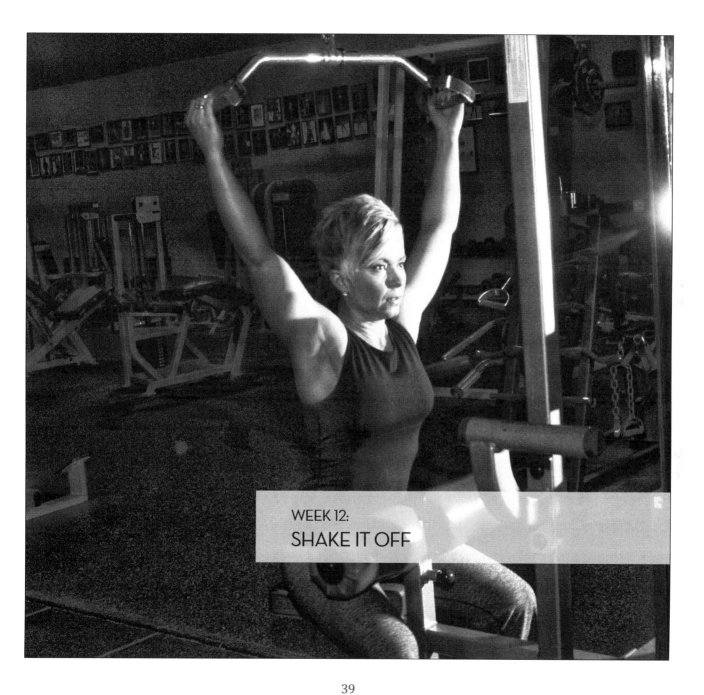

WEEK 12:
SHAKE IT OFF

My biggest struggle in life has always been my health. About 11 years ago, I was so sick I was certain my best years were not ahead of me. The doctors were not optimistic, my family looked at me with serious concern every time they came near me, and my dad took nearly a quarter of the year off work just to lay by my side. He presented the Bible to me and so did a few others. One day I decided I would give up. I was all alone in the house and I said, "I'm done, I don't want to live like this anymore. Instead of going through the process of healing and improving, I am ready to die." I accepted a terrible fate for myself. I had lost all hope and had no faith for a change. I turned on the television. While I laid on the couch about 98lbs, I turned on the television and saw pastor Jeff Perry. I didn't go to his church and didn't know him at all. He said, "Have you lost all hope, have you given up?" I said, "Yes sir, you bet I have." He said, "There is hope in Jesus. Receive him today, let him come in your heart and he will change your life." I did, and things have never been the same. I didn't give up. I read the scripture as if it were food

and medicine for my body. I spoke the scriptures out loud and declared it for my life. I was so sick I couldn't work at this time, so it became my full time job. I read Philippians 4:13, "I can do all things through Christ who strengthens me" daily and told myself this is my new language. Nothing will ever stop me from living a full life.

I shook off self-pity. I shook off bitterness and anger about being sick and why this happened to me. I shook off the hurt of understanding why I had to endure the pain. I may have been to hell and back, but God gave me a comeback. No matter what your past is, your best days are still out in front of you. I started studying nutrition. I removed all toxins from my life, chose to eat 100% organic food, and eliminated all gluten, dairy and soy from my diet. In this studying, I went from working ten years in the financial field - since I had graduated high school - to what I do now. Had I not endured the hardships and trials, I would not be where I am now doing what I do and changing lives each day. It was a stepping stone that took me to a higher place.

Stop dwelling on the past. I meet people and they tell me, "I have always struggled with food Debbie. I love to drink and party on the weekends Debbie. I can't stop myself from overeating Debbie. I don't have the time to do things the way you do them Debbie. I need a shortcut. I need a simplified version, an easy way to good health." Shake off the past and live in the present. Your best days are still ahead of you. Find something to stand on. I have my scripture, and you can have the same, but whatever it is make it your creed and dedicate yourself to it.

Don't let missed opportunities and past hardships or mistakes prevent you from living your best days now. Bury the past and resurrect yourself into a new life, a new future filled with hope and opportunity. Do it today. Your best days are out in front of you.

SAMPLE MENU

BREAKFAST
2 omega-3 organic egg omelet with
chopped mushroom, onion, spinach
to taste and top with picante
1 piece Ezekiel bread toasted with
omelet on top open face style

MID-MORNING SNACK
2 tbsp cooked whole steel cut oats
on top of
1 cup frozen blueberries thawed
2 tbsp sliced almonds with cinnamon
and Stevia to taste
1 scoop vanilla egg white protein with
water with 1/2 tsp cinnamon

LUNCH
7 oz Roasted Salmon on top of
3 cups fresh spinach with lemon
juice, apple cider
vinegar, and Stevia to taste

MID-AFTERNOON SNACK
1 apple
18 almonds
1 scoop vanilla egg white protein with
water and 1/2 tsp cinnamon

DINNER
5 oz ground bison mixed with
1/4 cup chili sauce
served on top of
3 cups Spaghetti Squash

DEBBIE'S MENU

4AM
6 egg white pancake
1 cup steamed green beans
1/2 cup mashed sweet potato

7AM
7 oz Grain-Free Turkey Meatloaf
3 cups baked green beans

10AM
6 egg whites
1 cup steamed green beans
1/2 cup mashed sweet potato

1PM
7 oz Grain-Free Turkey Meatloaf
3 cups baked green beans

4PM
6 egg whites
1 cup steamed green beans
1/2 cup mashed sweet potato

7PM
7 oz Grain-Free Turkey Meatloaf
3 cups baked green beans

BILL'S HEART HEALTHY MENU

BREAKFAST
3 egg whites, scrambled
3/4 scoop chocolate Jay Robb egg
white protein
1/2 banana
1/4 cup steel cut Irish oats

SNACK
1 Cinnamon Roll Larabar

LUNCH
6 oz Shredded BBQ Chicken
1/2 cup mashed sweet potato
2 cups mashed cauliflower

SNACK
2 containers applesauce
15 whole walnuts

DINNER
7 oz Agave Salmon
2 cups Roasted Broccoli
8 Roasted Carrots
2 tbsp brown rice

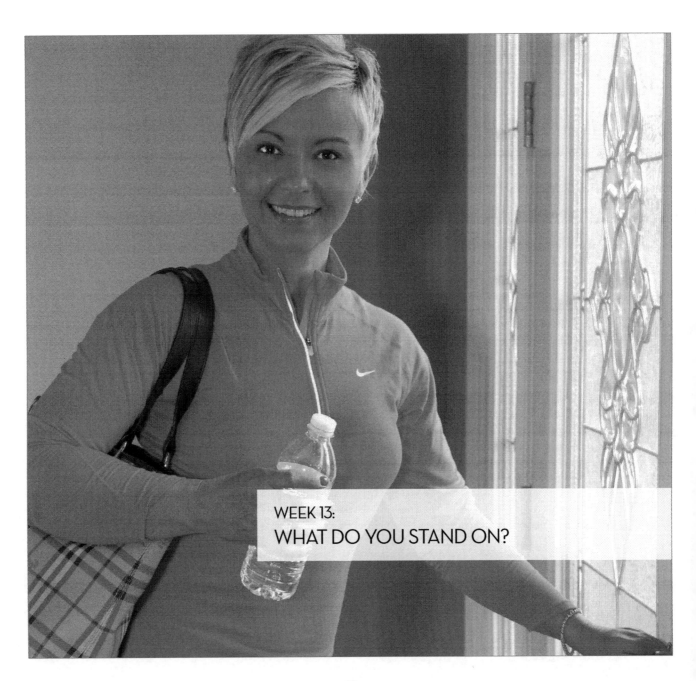

WEEK 13:
WHAT DO YOU STAND ON?

I can do all things through Christ who strengthens me. Philippians 4:13

Most people who know me are certain of what I stand on. I love this scripture. I have stood on it for years. I know I don't do things on my own, but with God I can do all things. When the chips are down or life is not going as I assumed it would, I stand on my foundation. My world cannot be shaken when I know I have this power behind me.

You may have taken a couple steps backward with your actions, but turn that around. Step out of the past and into the present. It's time for a comeback! Restore your mind and prepare yourself for victory. You can do this. You can do all things through Christ who strengthens you.

Whether your goals are weight loss, weight gain or health improvement, it will take drive and determination on your part to achieve them. If you have friends or family telling you to do things you shouldn't, don't listen to them!

Listen to me and collect a group of folks that support you and your goals. I am your friend and I want to see you victorious. True friends will be the same. I care about you, but most importantly, I care about your health. I want you to live life to the fullest! Choose life and health, not overindulgence and regret. This may seem hard, but it's equally as hard to live a life of regret after continually making poor choices.

Today is the day of no excuses, a fresh start. Keep the goals you want to achieve in front of you. See yourself fit and healthy. Speak that into your life always, not defeat. Accept a compliment with "Thanks" not with "Oh well I have a long way to go." Hold your head high and believe that this is the day the Lord has made. Rejoice and be glad in it! This image you place in front of you will set the framework of your life. When you choose an image of success for your life, the restrictions and limitations of defeated thinking will starve and no longer exist.

See your success. Schedule your success and live it! Determine the time each day that you can do your cardio. Determine the day each week that you can make your food. Stop the excuses. If I can do this, I promise you that you can. We are both busy. Stand on a firm foundation of health and wellness and refuse to allow anything else into your life. Your life and your spirit will be contagious.

Today is a new day. A fresh start. No more regret. Change your thoughts and change your world.

Have a wonderful week!
Do the work, no excuses.

SAMPLE MENU

BREAKFAST
2 egg omelette with 1 cup Roasted Broccoli chopped and topped with picante sauce
1/2 large grapefruit

MID-MORNING SNACK
1 Cherry Pie Larabar

LUNCH
5 oz Dijon Chicken
2 cups Roasted Cauliflower
1 cup steamed green beans

MID-AFTERNOON SNACK
1 scoop vanilla Jay Robb egg white protein blended with
1 cup mixed berries and
1 tbsp blackberry flax oil

DINNER
5 oz Chicken Wing Cutlets
2 cups Spaghetti Squash
1 cup sautéed peppers in olive oil

DEBBIE'S MENU

4AM
6 egg white pancake
1 cup steamed green beans
1/2 cup mashed sweet potato

7AM
6 oz Grain-Free Turkey Meatloaf
3 cups baked green beans

10AM
6 oz Grain-Free Turkey Meatloaf
1 cup steamed green beans
1/2 cup mashed sweet potato

1PM
6 egg white pancake
3 cups baked green beans

4PM
6 egg white pancake
1 cup steamed green beans
1/2 cup mashed sweet potato

7PM
6 oz Grain-Free Turkey Meatloaf
3 cups Roasted Broccoli

BILL'S HEART HEALTHY MENU

BREAKFAST
3 egg whites, scrambled
3/4 scoop chocolate Jay Robb egg white protein
1/2 banana
1/4 cup steel cut Irish oats

SNACK
1 Cinnamon Roll Larabar

LUNCH
6 oz Turkey Meatloaf
1/2 cup mashed sweet potato
2 cups mashed cauliflower

SNACK
2 containers applesauce
15 whole walnuts

DINNER
7 oz Turkey Meatloaf
2 cups Roasted Broccoli
8 Roasted Carrots
2 tbsp brown rice

TODAY IS THE DAY OF NO EXCUSES.
A FRESH START. KEEP THE GOALS YOU WANT TO ACHIEVE IN FRONT OF YOU. SEE YOURSELF FIT AND HEALTHY.

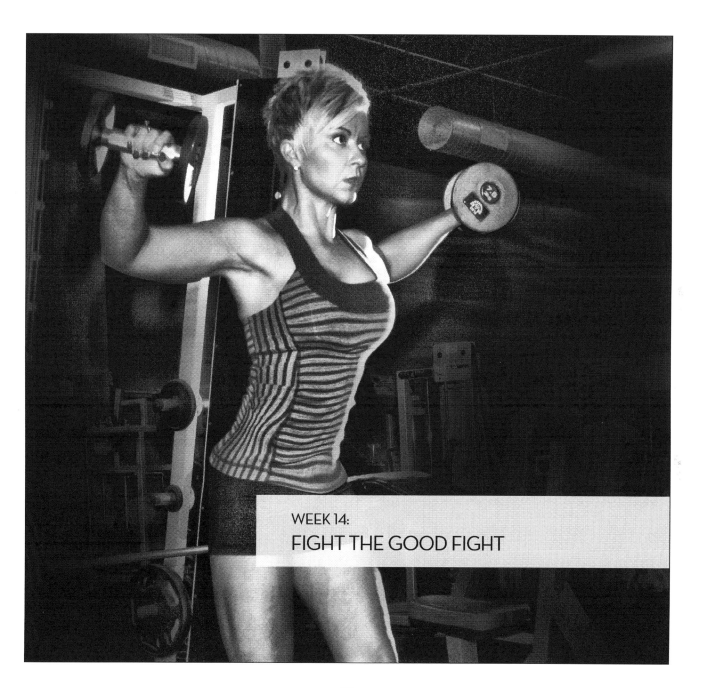

WEEK 14:
FIGHT THE GOOD FIGHT

"The mark of a true champion is knowing what battles to fight."
Joel Osteen

This couldn't be more true. I meet with people all day that are wasting their time fighting unnecessary battles. Someone has offended them, someone has bad-mouthed them, or someone doesn't believe in them. They are battling this out over and over in their mind trying to win, but they will never win. If someone has let you down and left you discouraged, don't waste your time fighting their battle. Run your own race and rise above it. If someone is bad-mouthing you behind your back, realize they are small-minded and you don't want to waste your time fighting a small-minded person. Rise above it and walk forward.

I have people tell me, "Debbie I can't eat like you or workout like you. I have kids, I have a busy job, my husband doesn't support me, I don't have the money or I lack the self discipline." Joel Osteen said, "Almost like a magnet, we draw in what we constantly think about. If we dwell on the lack in our life, we will continue to lack."

God wants you to soar like an eagle, to rise above defeated thinking and to excel in every area of your life. There will always be reasons why you are unsuccessful in changing your health. But before you hire me, join a gym, buy the groceries, invest in new shoes...First, change your attitude. Renew your mind and change the direction of your thinking.

Good health comes with work. It comes from a diligence in preparing your meals, continually making wise choices and not being affected by the pressure of your friends and family to do wrong. It comes from working out even when you don't have the time and don't want to make the effort. You may not want to be a professional athlete, but you do want to be healthy. Everyone does. Choose to have the attitude of a champion. Lay down the foundation of health by never giving into temptation and always being consistent with your workouts and meal preparation. You only have yourself to blame if you don't. Choose your battles wisely. Believe in yourself and live a life to please God, not others. When you do this, you will care less about what people think or say about you and more about doing what is right for you and your life.

SAMPLE MENU

BREAKFAST
Pumpkin Pancake topped with
1 tbsp almond butter, cinnamon
and Stevia
1 cup strawberries sliced

MID-MORNING SNACK
No Bake Apricot Bar

LUNCH
5 oz Ezekiel Bread Crumb
Chicken Cutlet
3 Zucchini Pancakes

MID-AFTERNOON SNACK
1 scoop chocolate Jay Robb egg
white protein blended with 1 cup
frozen cherries and 1 tbsp Barlean's
chocolate raspberry flax oil

DINNER
5 oz Pan-Seared Ezekiel Bread
Crusted Tilapia
1 cup steamed sugar snap snow peas
2 cups Roasted Broccoli

PRE-BEDTIME SNACK
1 scoop chocolate Jay Robb egg
white protein with 1 cup unsweetened almond milk

DEBBIE'S MENU

4AM
6 egg white pancake
1 cup steamed green beans
1/2 cup mashed sweet potato

7AM
1 scoop strawberry Jay Robb egg
white protein in water
1 tbsp strawberry-banana flax oil

9AM
1 scoop strawberry Jay Robb egg
white protein in water
1 tbsp strawberry-banana flax oil

11AM
5 oz Pan-Seared Chicken
1 cup steamed green beans with 1
tbsp chili sauce
1/2 cup mashed sweet potato

2PM
1 scoop strawberry Jay Robb egg
white protein in water
1 tbsp strawberry-banana flax oil

4PM
6 egg white pancake
1 cup steamed green beans
1/2 cup mashed sweet potato

7PM
5 oz Pan-Seared Chicken
3 cups steamed green beans

BILL'S HEART HEALTHY MENU

BREAKFAST
3 egg whites, scrambled
3/4 scoop chocolate Jay Robb egg
white protein
1/2 banana
1/4 cup steel cut Irish oats

SNACK
1 Cinnamon Roll Larabar

LUNCH
5 oz Pan-Seared Chicken
1/2 cup mashed sweet potato
2 cups mashed cauliflower

SNACK
2 containers applesauce
15 whole walnuts

DINNER
7 oz Agave Salmon
2 cups Roasted Broccoli
8 Roasted Carrots
2 tbsp brown rice

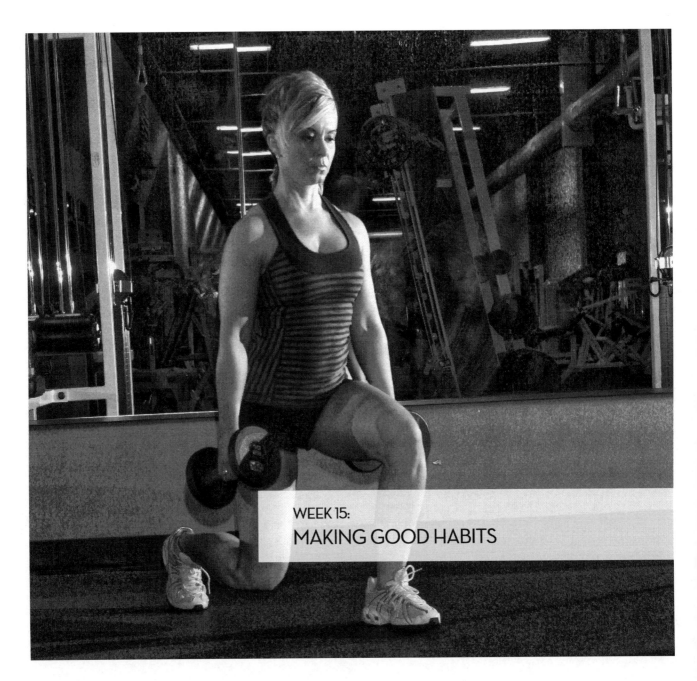

WEEK 15:
MAKING GOOD HABITS

"Your character is essentially the sum of your habits." Rick Warren

Growing up, I was raised in a home with parents of great moral character. They had great habits and strong convictions. My goal was to one day, be half the person my folks are. They love and respect each other and put their family before anyone.

As I have matured, I have found I am a creature of habit. I wake at the same time, work the same hours, workout at the exact same time every day, go home, make my food again, rest, sleep and then start over again. These are habits that get me through life, but these habits also make my character stronger. The fact that I get to bed on time, no matter who wants me to do what with them, allows me to perform at 100% for my clients. The fact that I do my workout at the same time each day makes it so that I am a living example for my clients and helps to keep my health on track. Preparing my food keeps my blood sugar stable, so I make sound decisions and walk in love to everyone I encounter.

Think over your habits. How are you spending your time? Is it how you really want your character to me molded? Think about the choices and decisions you are making each day. They don't always just affect you. Rick Warren also said, "Humility is not thinking less of yourself; it is thinking of yourself less." Try to remember your actions affect not only yourself, but all of those to whom your life is tied.

When we decide to get stuck in bad habits, our family and friends suffer the unfortunate consequences. They watch us become unhealthy, maybe deal with our bad attitudes or stress, and possibly have to pick up the pieces after our poor decisions go south.

No one is perfect, but creating a pattern of good habits of eating clean, exercising daily and taking time to renew your spirit is a great path to a positive life.

Be impeccable with your word and always do your best. Don't settle for second best. Don't lie to yourself or to anyone about why you can't do the right thing. You can always choose the right choice. Life is about choices. Don't settle for the easy route. Push through the challenges of life and receive the victory of a clear mind, great health, consistent energy patterns and a strong character. Be proud of who you are and what you value in life. The best way to do that is to be comfortable with your habits and your decisions. Mean what you say, and say what you mean.

A small reminder: When you see that cross, he took the nails for you. Forgiveness is granted as soon as you ask for it. We serve a God full of grace. Thank goodness he is full of mercy. If God can forgive you for your mistakes, then you must learn to forgive yourself.

Wake up tomorrow and talk yourself into having a great day.

SAMPLE MENU

BREAKFAST
3 egg whites scrambled with
2 oz ground bison topped with salsa
1 apple

MID-MORNING SNACK
1 No Bake Pumpkin Apricot bar

LUNCH
5 oz Hulkburger served onto piece of
chopped romaine lettuce with 1 tbsp
chili sauce on top
1 cup organic pumpkin mixed with
cinnamon and Stevia
2 cups roasted zucchini

MID-AFTERNOON SNACK
1 scoop vanilla Jay Robb egg white
blended with
1 tbsp lemon Barlean's fish oil
1 pear

DINNER
5 oz bison flank steak served over
1 cup Roasted Broccoli with
2 cups Spaghetti Squash

PRE-BEDTIME SNACK
1 cup unsweetened almond milk
mixed with
1/2 scoop chocolate Jay Robb egg
white protein

DEBBIE'S MENU

4AM
6 egg white pancake
1 cup steamed green beans
1/2 cup mashed sweet potato

7AM
1 scoop strawberry Jay Robb egg
white protein in water
1 tbsp strawberry-banana flax oil

9AM
1 scoop strawberry Jay Robb egg
white protein in water
1 tbsp strawberry-banana flax oil

11AM
5 oz shredded BBQ chicken
1 cup steamed green beans with
1 tbsp chili sauce
1/2 cup mashed sweet potato

2PM
1 scoop strawberry Jay Robb egg
white protein in water
1 tbsp strawberry-banana flax oil

7PM
5 oz shredded BBQ chicken
3 cups steamed green beans

BILL'S HEART HEALTHY MENU

BREAKFAST
3 egg whites, scrambled
3/4 scoop chocolate Jay Robb egg
white protein
1/2 banana
1/4 cup steel cut Irish oats

SNACK
1 Cinnamon Roll Larabar

LUNCH
5 oz shredded BBQ chicken
1/2 cup mashed sweet potato
2 cups mashed cauliflower

SNACK
2 containers applesauce
15 whole walnuts

DINNER
7 oz Agave Salmon
2 cups Roasted Broccoli
8 Roasted Carrots
2 tbsp brown rice

CREATING A PATTERN OF GOOD HABITS
OF EATING CLEAN, EXERCISING DAILY AND
TAKING TIME TO RENEW YOUR SPIRIT IS A
GREAT PATH TO A POSITIVE LIFE.

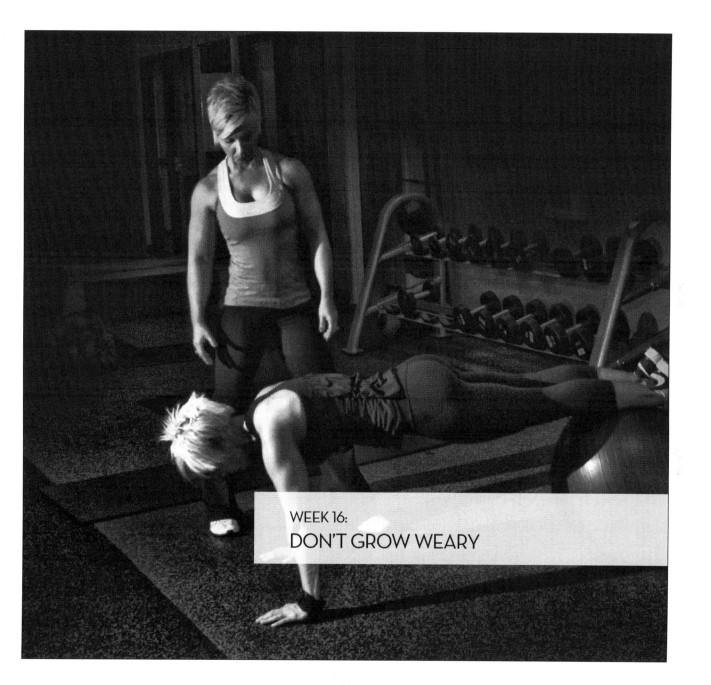

WEEK 16:
DON'T GROW WEARY

Let us not become weary in doing good, for at the proper time we will reap a harvest if we do not give up.
Galatians 6:9

This morning I read Joel Osteen who said, "All it takes is one *suddenly*. In a split second, with one touch of God's favor, everything can change." Sometimes we feel so overwhelmed in doing good. Making the chicken on Saturday instead of shopping, cooking the green beans every night instead of resting, drinking an iced tea when your friends are on their third round, waking before sunrise to do your workout when everyone else you know is nursing their hangover in bed, choosing to think clean, eat clean and live clean even when it's not the popular choice. It's easy to grow weary in doing good.

Don't miss your harvest. The harvest is near. When is your "*suddenly*" coming? Is it the day the doctor takes you off your medication? Is it when your spouse says wow, you look outstanding? Is it when you run that mile, and instead of dying to get to the finish line, you're ready to run one more? Is it the day that wayward friend or family member who lacks motivation, confidence, and discipline seeks you out for advice because you are an example of inspiration and motivation without ever discussing it with them?

When will your "*suddenly*" come? Open your eyes to the fact that a "*suddenly*" will come for you everyday. Your harvest is here for you to reach out and grab it. Don't give up just short of the prize! Fight! Fight for what you want in life. Health is achievable by everyone. Simple steps can change everything. Don't make excuses anymore. Today is the day for your harvest. Live it. Clean eating, cardio and strength training will change your life. What will change it even more is clean living and clean thinking. Change the filter in your mind that keeps reminding you of your failures, shortcomings and insecurities. You have the remote control! Change the channel in your mind. Remind yourself you're amazing, you're victorious, you're healthy and you're driven. All of this can be yours if you don't grow weary. Don't miss your harvest. Open your eyes today and talk yourself into having a great day. Suddenly, I think favor will come your way.

Have a wonderful week,
Deb

REMIND YOURSELF YOU'RE AMAZING, YOU'RE VICTORIOUS, YOU'RE HEALTHY, AND YOU'RE DRIVEN!

ALL OF THIS CAN BE YOURS IF YOU DON'T GROW WEARY.

SAMPLE MENU

BREAKFAST
Equal Parts Protein Pancake

MID-MORNING SNACK
1 scoop vanilla egg white protein
mixed with
1 cup unsweetened almond milk and
1/2 tsp cinnamon
1 pear sliced and heated in the
microwave for 90 seconds topped
with 18 walnuts

LUNCH
1 bowl Bison Beef Stew

MID-AFTERNOON SNACK
1 cup organic goat's milk yogurt
topped with
1 1/2 cups frozen organic mixed berries and
2 tbsp sliced almonds

DINNER
5 oz Lemon Chicken
2 cups Roasted Broccoli
1 sliced tomato drizzled with
balsamic vinegar

DEBBIE'S MENU

4AM
6 egg white pancake
1 cup steamed green beans
1/2 cup mashed sweet potato

7AM
5 oz Grain-Free Turkey Meatloaf
3 cups steamed green beans

10AM
1 scoop strawberry Jay Robb egg
white protein in water
1 cup steamed green beans
1/2 cup mashed sweet potato

1PM
5 oz Grain-Free Turkey Meatloaf
3 cups steamed green beans

4PM
6 egg white pancake
1 cup steamed green beans
1/2 cup mashed sweet potato

7PM
5 oz Grain-Free Turkey Meatloaf
3 cups steamed green beans

BILL'S HEART HEALTHY MENU

BREAKFAST
3 egg whites, scrambled
3/4 scoop chocolate Jay Robb egg
white protein
1/2 banana
1/4 cup steel cut Irish oats

SNACK
1 Cinnamon Roll Larabar

LUNCH
7 oz Turkey Meatloaf
1/2 cup mashed sweet potato
2 cups mashed cauliflower
4 Roasted Carrots

SNACK
2 containers applesauce
15 whole walnuts

DINNER
7 oz Agave Salmon
2 cups Roasted Broccoli
4 Roasted Carrots
2 tbsp brown rice

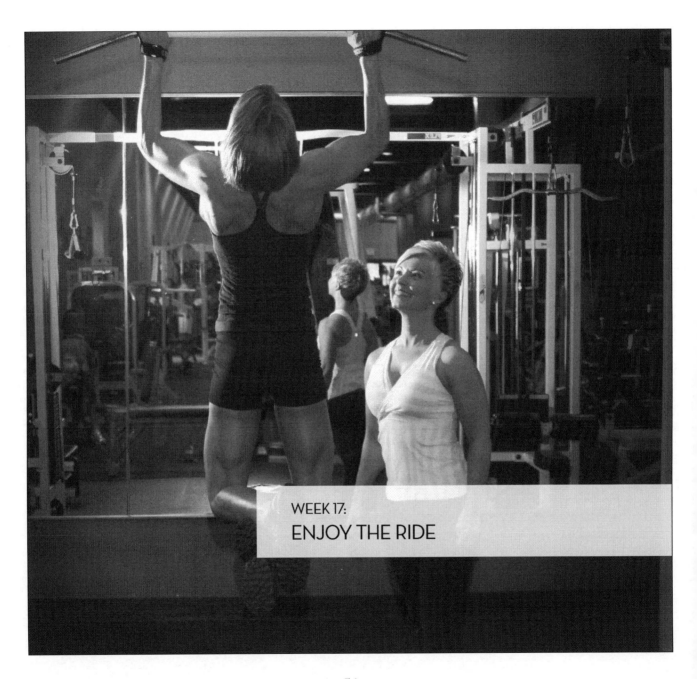

WEEK 17:
ENJOY THE RIDE

You don't have to wait for life - your job, your weight, your marriage - to be perfect to be happy. Even if you're not where you want to be, you're on your way to where you want to go.

How many of you have forgotten about the ride? We are so concerned with the destination that we forget to enjoy the ride. My clients approach me all of the time with, "Debbie, I have to lose this weight before I am 40. I have to have a perfect shape before my show. I have to get into that dress before my party." But what about the ride? Joel Osteen says, "Life flies by, so don't waste precious time being worried. This is the day God wants you to choose to be happy."

I agree that your future and your goals need to govern your thoughts, and the preparation to reaching those goals must consume your time. However, I ask you to stop and take a minute to enjoy where you are in life. If you're training for a show, trying to lose weight for a special event, or losing weight you have needed to lose for a lifetime, look in the mirror and realize you look the best you have ever looked and will continue to look better with each passing day.

It is a simple truth that happiness is a choice, so we each need to choose to be happy. Maybe you're not at your goal yet, but instead of worrying that you won't make it to that goal, choose to be happy along the ride. Do the work and put in the time. Clean eating, clean living and clean thinking will get you there. Constant worry about tomorrow combined with a constant defeated attitude will only hold you back and certainly make for a rough ride.

Joel Osteen also says, "We all have difficulties and challenges. But if we allow those circumstances to dictate our happiness, we risk missing out on God's abundant life he intends for us." Don't allow past failures and mistakes to dictate the path of your future. Stay motivated toward your goals and never give up. However, don't forget to enjoy the path to success. Each day is a blessing. Choose to enjoy the ride; the path to success is covered with failures, but those failures equal great opportunity for growth.

Good luck to you this week as you work to reach your goals. I am blessed to have many of you as my clients. For the rest of you, I pray that your life is filled with happiness.

Have a blessed week.
Debbie

INSTEAD OF WORRYING THAT YOU WON'T MAKE IT TO THAT GOAL, CHOOSE TO BE HAPPY ALONG THE RIDE.

SAMPLE MENU

BREAKFAST
Sweet Potato Pancake with
1 tsp almond butter spread on top

MID-MORNING SNACK
1 1/2 cup berries, 1 tbsp crumbled
goat cheese on top
1 tsp Agave all warmed together for
20 seconds

LUNCH
5 oz Bison Roast, large spinach salad
with tomatoes, red onion, red pepper
1 tbsp olive oil, 1 tbsp apple cider
vinegar, garlic powder, pepper to
taste and 1/2 packet of Stevia

MID-AFTERNOON SNACK
1 pear and 1 apple chopped and
warmed for 1 minute 30 seconds.
Top with 2 tbsp chopped pecans,
cinnamon and Stevia to taste

DINNER
7 oz Lemon Pepper Grilled
Crunch Salmon
2 cups Roasted Broccoli
1 cup roasted red pepper

PRE-BEDTIME SNACK
1 scoop chocolate egg white protein
with 1 tbsp chocolate raspberry flax oil
and 1 cup unsweetened almond milk

DEBBIE'S MENU

4AM
Sweet Potato Pancake
1 cup baked green beans

7AM
4 oz Bison Roast
3 cups baked green beans

10AM
Sweet Potato Pancake
1 cup baked green beans

1PM
1 scoop strawberry Jay Robb egg
white protein with
1/2 cup unsweetened almond milk
1 tsp Barlean's strawberry banana
flax oil
3 cups baked green beans

4PM
Sweet Potato Pancake
1 cup baked green beans

7PM
5 oz Lemon Pepper Grilled
Crunch Salmon
3 cups baked green beans

BILL'S HEART HEALTHY MENU

BREAKFAST
3 egg whites, scrambled
3/4 scoop chocolate Jay Robb egg
white protein
1/2 banana
1/4 cup steel cut Irish oats

SNACK
1 Cinnamon Roll Larabar

LUNCH
5 oz BBQ Shredded Chicken
1 1/2 cup mashed cauliflower
3/4 cup mashed sweet potato

SNACK
1/2 cup unsweetened 365 organic
applesauce and
15 whole walnuts

DINNER
6 oz Agave Salmon
2 cups Roasted Broccoli recipe
2 tbsp brown rice sprinkled on top of
broccoli and
6 roasted baby carrots
2 tbsp brown rice

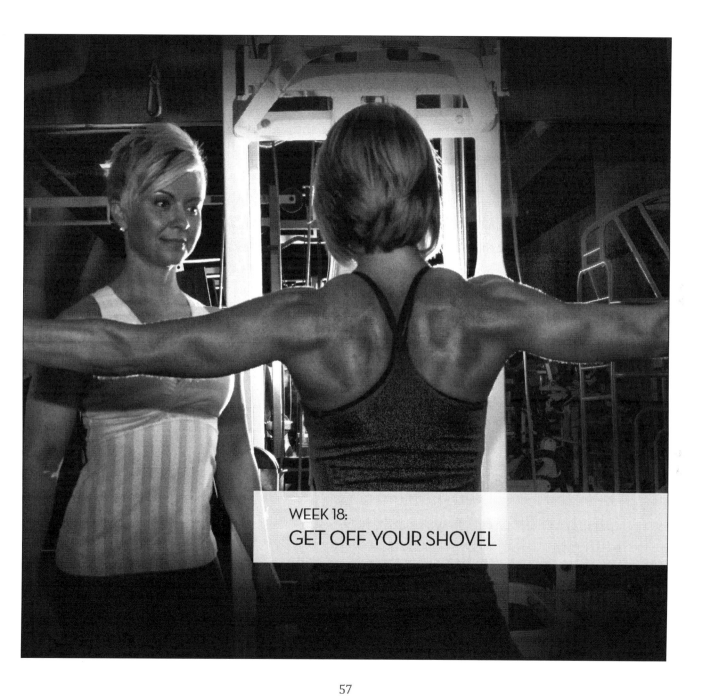

WEEK 18:
GET OFF YOUR SHOVEL

Whatever your hand finds to do, do it with all your might. Ecclesiastes 9:10

Today I was reading and Joel Osteen said, "If you are digging a ditch, don't spend half the day leaning on your shovel; do your work with excellence and enthusiasm." How many of us are leaning on our shovel? How many will say, "I will get to my cardio later today. I will start eating clean tomorrow, next week, or next month. Until then, I will rest here on my shovel."
Step out of excuses! Put that shovel in your hands and start digging.

Today is the day and this hour is the time. This is your life - your heart, lungs, liver and kidneys - we are talking about. What will happen when caring for your body has been prolonged for too long? Will we visit you in the hospital? I hope not! Is it really worth it to you to have that meal instead of cooking and preparing clean food? Is it worth it to go out drinking with your friends instead of getting a full night's rest to restore your body?

Is it worth it to lean on that shovel instead of making the time to do your cardio and workout?

If you can't get out of a hole, then call me or some other professional. Schedule an appointment to change your life. Take one of these free meal plans, cook them for the week, and see how good you can feel! Schedule an appointment with a trainer and become accountable for your nutrition and exercise. Seek help at least until you can motivate yourself on your own.

This week, get your grip back on life. It will pass you by before you know it. You don't need something extraordinary to happen in your life to live in faith, joy, peace and passion. Clean your mind and change your thinking. Flip from the page of the old way of thinking to a new page. Get a vision for a better and healthier way of living today. Grab a hold of that shovel and start digging your way to a new life of health and happiness.

No one is too deep in anything. Everyone can see improvements in their situation. If you will stay in faith and not lose passion for life, I promise your life will bless you each new day. Banish thoughts of defeat - I'm too tired, too hurt, too defeated, too broke - from your mind. Give up on that way of thinking; it has gotten you nowhere.

The three C's of living are clean eating, clean thinking and clean living. Make it your motto today. I will eat clean, I will think clean thoughts of victory and favor, not of defeat. Finally, choose to follow the path of clean living - the right path for you, your family, and your body - no matter how hard. Choose to exercise. You can do all of this. It just takes one day to start changing your habits. Start it today.

Have a great week!
God Bless, Deb

SAMPLE MENU

BREAKFAST
Apple Cinnamon Pancake
Top with 1 tbsp of almond butter

MID-MORNING SNACK
1 1/2 cup berries
1 tbsp crumbled goat cheese on top
1 tsp agave nectar all warmed
together for 20 seconds

LUNCH
5 oz Baked Chicken on top of
2 tbsp brown rice
1 1/2 cups Roasted Broccoli

MID-AFTERNOON SNACK
1 scoop chocolate egg white protein
1 tbsp natural peanut butter and
1 1/2 banana

DINNER
5 oz Lemon Garlic Roasted
Turkey Breast
2 cups Spaghetti Squash
8 spears of roasted Balsamic
Asparagus

DEBBIE'S MENU

4AM
Sweet Potato Pancake
1 cup baked green beans

7AM
4 oz Bison Roast
3 cups baked green beans

10AM
Sweet Potato Pancake
1 cup baked green beans

1PM
1 scoop vanilla Jay Robb egg white
protein with
1/2 cup unsweetened almond milk
3/4 tbsp Barlean's strawberry banana
flax oil
2 cups baked green beans

4PM
Sweet Potato Pancake
1 cup baked green beans

7PM
5 oz Lemon Pepper Grilled
Crunch Salmon
2 cups baked green beans

BILL'S HEART HEALTHY MENU

BREAKFAST
3 egg whites, scrambled
3/4 scoop chocolate Jay Robb egg
white protein
1/2 banana
1/4 cup steel cut Irish oats

SNACK
1 Cinnamon Roll Larabar

LUNCH
5 oz BBQ Shredded Chicken
1 1/2 cup mashed cauliflower
3/4 cup mashed sweet potato

AFTERNOON SNACK
1/2 cup unsweetened 365 organic
applesauce
15 whole walnuts

DINNER
6 oz Agave Salmon
2 cups Roasted Broccoli
2 tbsp brown rice sprinkled on top
of broccoli
6 roasted baby carrots

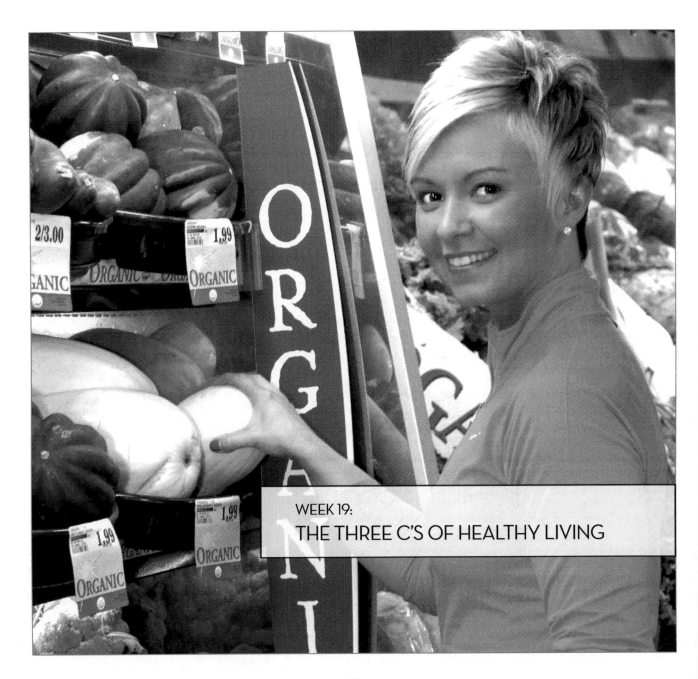

WEEK 19:
THE THREE C'S OF HEALTHY LIVING

Clean eating, clean thinking and clean living.

Each day I wake up and pray that God will guide my steps, my choices and my words. I pray that in an imperfect world, he will give me the strength and courage to represent his goodness and mercy to each person I encounter. During the 41 days my dad was in the hospital, I spent hours in prayer. I prayed Psalm 91 out loud over him and declared each word of it as a victory for him and expected a result. A couple days after his most challenging surgery, he had one of his hardest days and I was there alone for the better part of the day. We just kept reading it, declaring it, and believing it would come to pass.

It did!

When I send the weekly e-mails and post my messages, I hope someone receives them and is blessed by them. I expect God to provide just the right touch to motivate someone to start living better and reaching for new, healthier heights with their life. I expect that if my faith is contagious,

then my enthusiasm toward healthy living will also be contagious and as a result, many more people will step up and take their lives to the next level.

As we met with the hospital dietitian, I was almost frightened for my father's future. Each member of the staff was at least 30lbs overweight, including the doctors. None of them had really found the answer. As I read the ingredients to the prepared meal replacement shakes they expected him to take three times a day, I realized he was going to end up right back in the hospital in no time. That is what motivated me to start posting the meal plans and messages, then write this cookbook. Eventually I started preparing Dad's food on my own and went outside the boundaries of the food pyramid.

There are so many misconceptions about food. If you are dieting and not losing weight, still on your medication or not feeling your best, then please hire a professional to help you. Not just any professional, someone who has experienced it themselves or who

has five to twenty years' experience in working with clients and a proven track record for success. When I look at a successful nutritionist or trainer's track record, I want to see if their clients keep the weight off. Do they put it back on a year later because they can't keep up with it? A quality trainer and nutritionist works on the whole problem. They teach you clean eating, clean thinking and clean living. They teach it in a way that is long-term and life-altering. These suggestions should be applicable for a lifetime. They should produce results over time not suddenly. They should help you to eliminate the need for medication and have you feeling healthier than ever before.

I've been working out in a gym since I was in the fourth grade with my father. I did gymnastics at the YMCA and worked out in the weight room with my dad. In junior high, we moved to George Turner's gym in South County. I also took four years of body building in high school. Then, we moved to Powerhouse with Tom Hobbs as the owner and have been with Roger and his gang ever since. I have worked out at several Gold's Gyms, Lifetime Fitnesses and 24 Hour Fitnesses across the country. I know and understand what it takes to make a gym successful. I also know the difference between a life-changing trainer and nutritionist.

Hire someone who lives the trade. They don't have to look like a body builder; they simply need to live a healthy life. They need to present themselves professionally; their focus should be entirely on you and your success. They must have the tools to get you where you need to go. Even more importantly than all of this, they must speak words of faith to you. Not gossip, not defeat. Instead, they should build you up each session and design a path for success. They should never give up on you, no matter how many times you fail. They must represent a creed and stick to that pattern of beliefs, not conform to other beliefs in order to please you or others around them. I live this profession. I may not look like a body builder, but that's because I'm not one. I am a 36-year-old woman with Hashimoto's Disease who has found a way to be victorious even through difficult circumstances. I love my clients like they are members of my family and most of my clients have been with me for three to six years. Find someone who is passionate about eating clean. Eating whole, real foods not loaded with preservatives. There are no shortcuts to a healthy life. Find someone who has clean thinking. You want someone who speaks success into your life and shows you the path of victorious living, not defeated living. Finally, find someone who lives clean and represents themselves and their company professionally. This is not a job to me, it is my passion. Search and find someone like that. I have a whole staff of them! Clean living means regular strength training and cardio. It means avoiding a life of overindulgence and possessing the mental strength and fortitude to choose healthy choices for a better life, no matter the circumstances.

Finally, find someone who is an advocate of health.

If you don't believe in yourself, then change it! Start today; believe that you can lose this weight, drop that medication and change your life. The barrier is in your mind.

Have a blessed week.
DEB

THREE C'S OF HEALTHY LIVING CLEAN EATING, CLEAN THINKING AND CLEAN LIVING.

SAMPLE MENU

BREAKFAST
Blueberry Banana Pancake
Top with 1 tbsp ground almond
butter and 1/2 cup blueberries

MID-MORNING SNACK
1 cup 2% greek yogurt
1/2 scoop chocolate Jay Robb egg
white protein blended with
8 frozen strawberries

LUNCH
2 ladles full of Bison Chili

MID-AFTERNOON SNACK
20 almonds
1 pear

DINNER
5 oz Grilled Bison Burger
4 pieces of thick-sliced home-grown
tomatoes topped with 1 tsp olive oil,
salt, pepper, garlic powder and sliced
red onion

DEBBIE'S MENU

4 AM
6 egg whites
1/2 cup pumpkin
1 cup green beans with 1/2 tsp olive oil

7 AM
4 oz Bison Roast
2 cups steamed green beans,
1 tsp olive oil

10AM
6 egg whites
1/2 cup pumpkin
1 cup green beans, 1/2 tsp olive oil

1PM
4 oz Bison Roast
2 cups steamed green beans, 1 tsp
olive oil

4PM
6 egg whites
2 cups steamed green beans
1 tsp olive oil

7PM
4 oz BBQ Shredded Chicken
2 cups steamed green beans with
1 tsp olive oil

BILL'S HEART HEALTHY MENU

BREAKFAST
3 egg whites, scrambled
3/4 scoop chocolate Jay Robb egg
white protein
1/2 banana
1/4 cup steel cut Irish oats

MID MORNING SNACK
15 walnuts

LUNCH
5 oz BBQ Shredded Chicken
1 cup mashed cauliflower
3/4 cup mashed sweet potato
6 roasted baby carrots

AFTERNOON SNACK
1 Cinnamon Roll Larabar

DINNER
6 oz Agave Salmon
2 cups Roasted Broccoli
2 tbsp brown rice sprinkled on top
of broccoli
6 roasted baby carrots

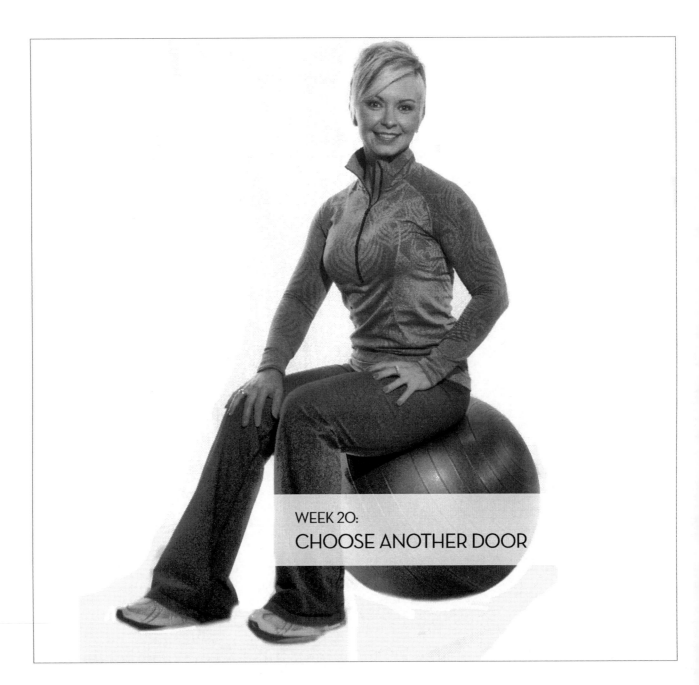

WEEK 20:
CHOOSE ANOTHER DOOR

What door did you walk out of today? The door of defeat or the door of success? Are you expecting goodness and mercy to follow you through your day today, or failure and defeat? How many of you are waking up this morning walking through the door of past mistakes, of overindulging in food or drinks, of disappointment in yourself and your decisions? Today is a new day. Yesterday is long gone. It will never be out in front of you again, so choose another door. Take a step to the right and walk through the door of change, success, health and favor. Decide today that your eating will be clean, your mind will be free of defeated thinking, your choices will improve and your health will be considered above all else.

Put your tennis shoes on before you hit that chair. Take a walk around the block; it is a beautiful day to be alive. I have a network of people I minister to daily and I wish I could tell you how rough some of these people have it. They can't breathe right, swallow right, see right, they have blood sugar issues, or heart issues and all they pray for is to be healthy enough to do exactly what you are fully capable of doing daily. Make the choice today to step out of a life of defeat driven by poor choices and into a life of health and favor. I don't care if you have 20lbs or 100lbs to lose; get someone involved in your victory. Hire someone to help you achieve this.

Life can hit you like a ton of bricks sometimes. As you become more positive, more motivated and more successful, people will always try to find a way to criticize you and your methods. Who cares? Let them. Who needs them anyway? Anyone who spends their time trying to prove their worth by degrading someone else is only proving their own ignorance and insecurity.

As you go through this journey toward a healthy life, don't let these bumps derail you. Let the unhappy, critical people be the way they are. Walk in love in front of them. Endure hardship as a soldier and plant the seed of your success in them by walking in love in front of them.

Never ever let it get you down. Never let your critics get the best of you. Don't live to please your critics; live to please God, and I can guarantee you a happy life.

SAMPLE MENU

BREAKFAST
1 piece Egg White French Toast
1 cup plain greek yogurt
1 scoop strawberry Jay Robb egg
white protein blended

MID-MORNING SNACK
6 egg white pancake
1 apple
20 almonds

LUNCH
5 oz Lemon-Garlic Roasted
Turkey Breast
1/2 cup mashed sweet potato
1 cup greek yogurt combined with
1 chopped and peeled cucumber and
1/2 of a small chopped onion. Blend
well in blender or food processor
and add sea salt and pepper

MID-AFTERNOON SNACK
1 cup berries
1 scoop vanilla Jay Robb egg white
protein blended
1 tbsp blueberry pomegranate flax oil

DINNER
5 oz Hulkburger
2 cups Roasted Broccoli
1 cup roasted carrots

DEBBIE'S MENU

4AM
5 oz BBQ Shredded Chicken
1/2 cup pumpkin
1 cup steamed green beans with
1/2 tsp olive oil

7AM
4 oz Bison Roast
2 cups steamed green beans with 1
tsp olive oil

10AM
5 oz BBQ Shredded Chicken
1/2 cup pumpkin
1 cup steamed green beans with
1/2 tsp olive oil

1PM
4 oz Bison Roast
2 cups steamed green beans with
1 tsp olive oil

4PM
5 oz BBQ Shredded Chicken
1/2 cup pumpkin
1 cup steamed green beans with
1/2 tsp olive oil

7PM
4 oz Bison Roast
2 cups steamed green beans with
1 tsp olive oil

BILL'S HEART HEALTHY MENU

BREAKFAST
3 egg whites scrambled
3/4 scoop chocolate Jay Robb egg
white protein
1/2 banana
1/4 cup steel cut Irish oats

MID SNACK
15 walnuts

LUNCH
5 oz BBQ Shredded Chicken
1 cup mashed cauliflower
3/4 cup mashed sweet potato
6 roasted baby carrots

AFTERNOON SNACK
1 Cinnamon Roll Larabar

DINNER
6 oz Agave Salmon
2 cups Roasted Broccoli
2 tbsp brown rice sprinkled on
top of broccoli
6 roasted baby carrots

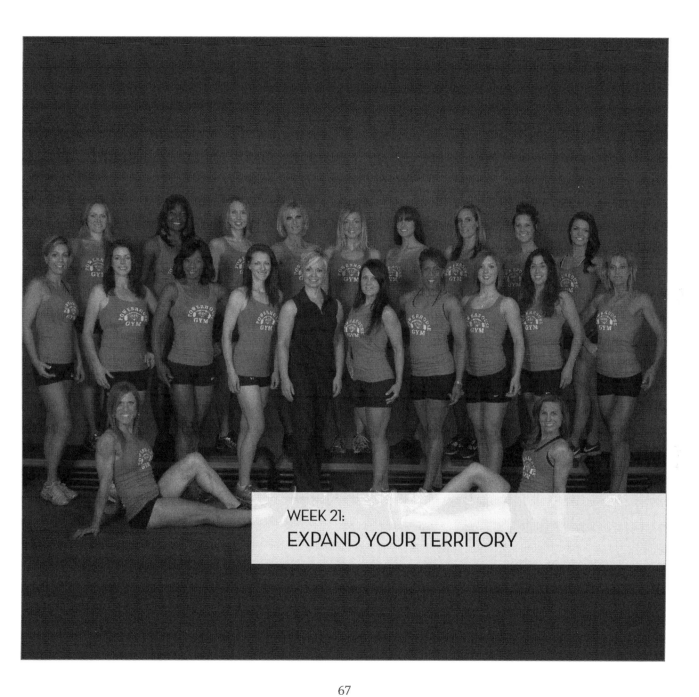

WEEK 21:
EXPAND YOUR TERRITORY

What boundaries have you placed on your life? If you wake up daily accepting and expecting the worst to happen, then you're navigating directly towards a lifetime of failure. I meet with many people who tell me, "Debbie, I have tried all the diets out there, all the programs available. I've been on them all, but I never complete them. I always give up." I get told they don't have enough time, they have a family, a busy job, too many social functions or are just too lazy. These boundaries have driven them to and through consistent failure.

If you continue to fail to lose weight, then I suggest stepping off of your current path and hiring a professional to help you organize and redirect your path. When looking for a professional, choose someone who lives the trade. Does this person walk the walk or just talk the talk? Find a professional who will sit with you and discover your mistakes and who will have the courage to force you to see your hindrances and confront them. Find a person who is positive and brings good energy to everyone, who does not pass judgment on others nor is critical and gossipy. You need to be surrounded by positive energy and to close the door once and for all to those who are bringing you down.

When I take on a client, I climb into their world. I ride the wave of expectancies they have for themselves. When they are weak, I am strong. When I am not there for them, I provide them with the ammunition to fight their battle alone. I give them motivation to believe in themselves. I train them to redirect their thoughts into a clean pattern of thinking. I provide tools to do a correct routine for their body when they are on their own, and skills to shop and prepare correctly to keep their mind and body running efficiently.

Clean thinking means expecting the best of your life. The past is the past. Put your failures, to rest and increase your territory. Move outside of the boundaries you have set for your life. You have continued to remind yourself of past failures so you comfortably allow yourself to live within the boundaries of those failures. Step out in faith and believe in yourself; believe that God not only has more in store for you, but that he expects more out of you. Choose to live a limitless life. You can do all things through Christ who strengthens you. Don't talk yourself out of a fresh start. Don't convince yourself you're going to fail if you try again. The solution is right around the corner.

SAMPLE MENU

BREAKFAST
1 cup goat's milk yogurt
3/4 scoop vanilla Jay Robb egg white
protein
1 cup frozen organic mixed berries
thawed
Blend and enjoy chilled

MID-MORNING SNACK
20 almonds
4 dried apricots

LUNCH
4 oz Pan-Seared Chicken
on top of 2 cups sautéed spinach
1 cup Spaghetti Squash with
1 tbsp chili sauce

MID-AFTERNOON SNACK
1 apricot No Bake Protein Bar

DINNER
5 oz Bison Mini Meatloaf
2 cups Roasted Broccoli

LATE SNACK
1 cup unsweetened almond milk
1/2 scoop strawberry Jay Robb egg
white protein

DEBBIE'S MENU

4AM
6 egg whites
1/2 baked sweet potato

7AM
4 oz Bison Chuck Roast
2 cups baked green beans

10AM
6 egg whites
1/2 baked sweet potato plain

1PM
4 oz Bison Sirloin roast
2 cups green beans

4PM
6 egg whites with
2 cups baked green beans

7PM
5 oz BBQ Shredded Chicken with
2 cups baked green beans

BILL'S HEART HEALTHY MENU

BREAKFAST
3 egg whites scrambled
3/4 scoop chocolate Jay Robb egg
white protein
1/2 banana
1/4 cup steel cut Irish oats

MID SNACK
15 walnuts

LUNCH
5 oz BBQ Shredded Chicken
1 cup mashed cauliflower
3/4 cup mashed sweet potato
6 roasted baby carrots

AFTERNOON SNACK
1 Cinnamon Roll Larabar

DINNER
6 oz Agave Salmon
2 cups Roasted Broccoli
2 tbsp brown rice sprinkled on top
of broccoli
6 roasted baby carrots

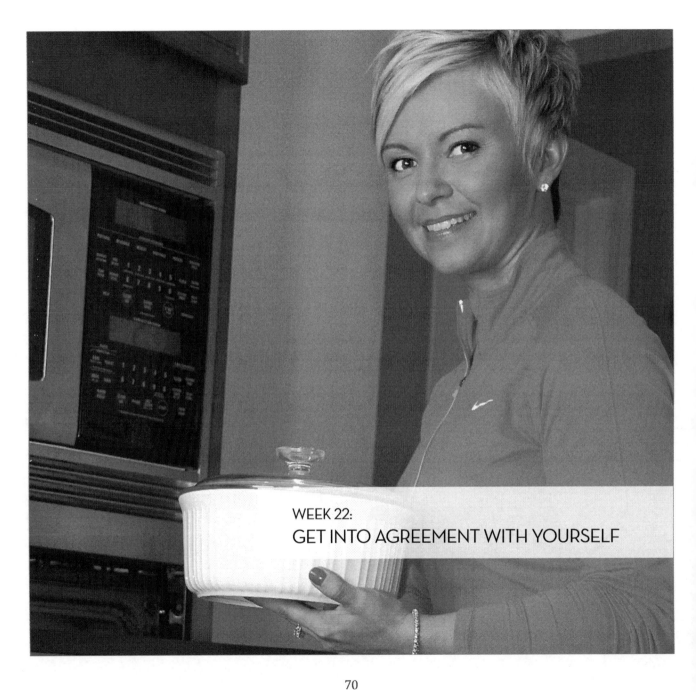

WEEK 22:
GET INTO AGREEMENT WITH YOURSELF

Years ago, I found myself weak-minded and overwhelmed with concern over what others might think of me. I worried if I was skinny enough, if my clothes were pressed well enough, if my house was clean enough, if my car was nice enough, if I upset someone, or if someone didn't like me. It was a life full of nonsense. As I started to explore my faith, I realized the only opinion I needed to care about was that of God. Not my boss, not my husband, not my family, not my friends and not my neighbors. Suddenly, as I read the scriptures, I would feel the pressures of life lighten with each new day. I would wake up and pray that God would guide my steps each day.

I started to generate a creed for my life similar to the military or a code of ethics. I decided I would follow this creed. I was raised this way but as I grew older, I grew further and further away from it. When my folks instilled this code into me as a child, they had a purpose. The purpose behind it was living a faith-filled life. When you choose to please and seek God first in life, everything else just seems to fall into place. When you choose to fulfill your own desires or the desires of others, you live a life lacking in peace and full of discontent.

Create your own creed today. Mine originates in the Bible and was passed onto me from my parents. I read daily to enrich my walk in life. I am in no way free from failure. I have made millions of mistakes, but I can say that I now live a life free from worry about what people think and say about me. There will always be haters in life. They hate on you because they don't like their own life. If they did, they would be far too busy to hate on you. Don't waste your time trying to win them over. Invest your time in the three C's of healthy living: clean eating, clean thinking and clean living.

Don't let stress sabotage your health and your weight loss goals.

You're in control.

SAMPLE MENU

BREAKFAST
Baked Bison Omelet
1 cup fresh berries

MID-MORNING SNACK
1 cherry chocolate No Bake
Protein Bar

LUNCH
5 oz Kickin' Chicken
2 cups Roasted Broccoli
2 tbsp brown rice on top of broccoli

MID-AFTERNOON SNACK
20 almonds
1 Pink Lady apple

DINNER
6 oz Fiesta Lime Tilapia
1 cup baked green beans
2 cups Spaghetti Squash

DEBBIE'S MENU

4 AM
6 egg whites
1/4 cup pumpkin
1 1/2 cup green beans with 1 tsp olive oil

7 AM
4 oz Bison Roast
2 cups steamed green beans with
1 tsp olive oil

10AM
6 egg whites
1/4 cup pumpkin
1 1/2 cup green beans with 1 tsp olive oil

1PM
4 oz Bison Roast
2 cups steamed green beans with
1 tsp olive oil

4PM
6 egg whites
2 cup steamed green bean with
1 tsp olive oil

7PM
4 oz BBQ Shredded Chicken
2 cup steamed green beans with
1 tsp olive oil

BILL'S HEART HEALTHY MENU

BREAKFAST
3 egg whites scrambled
3/4 scoop chocolate Jay Robb egg
white protein
1/2 banana
1/4 cup steel cut Irish oats

MID MORNING SNACK
15 walnuts

LUNCH
5 oz BBQ Shredded Chicken
1 cup mashed cauliflower
3/4 cup mashed sweet potato
6 roasted baby carrots

AFTERNOON SNACK
1 Cinnamon Roll Larabar

DINNER
6 oz Agave Salmon
2 cups Roasted Broccoli
2 tbsp brown rice sprinkled on
top of broccoli
6 roasted baby carrots

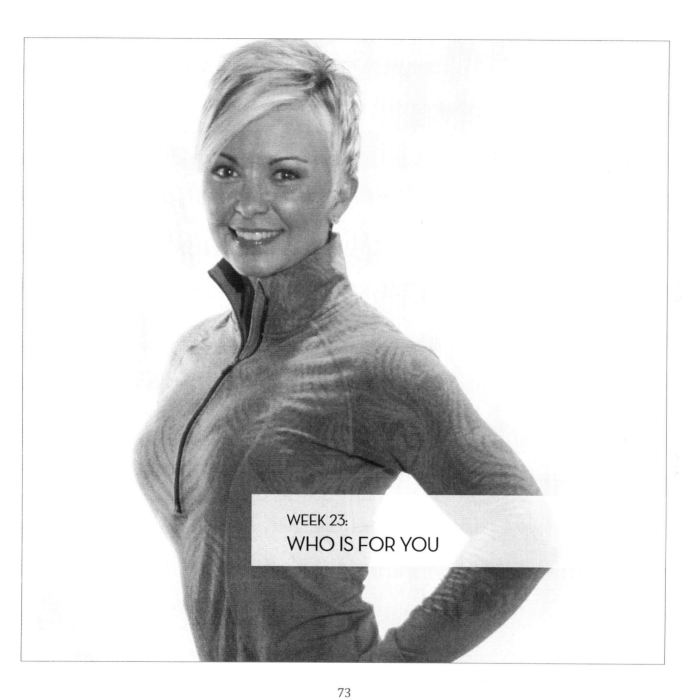

WEEK 23:
WHO IS FOR YOU

"God will always bring the right people into your life, but you have to let the wrong people walk away. The right people will never show up if you don't clear out the wrong people. If you stay open, God will give you people who are not just WITH you, but FOR you."
- Joel Osteen

This statement is so true. I meet with so many clients who are frustrated with themselves because they've allowed others to deter them from their goals. They continue to spend time with people who defeat them instead of support them. They feel obligated to someone who refuses to see the importance of their exercise regimen, clean eating and new approach to health. These clients continue to feel overwhelmed by the choice of being the new person they want to become or being held back by the people who want to defeat them.

If you allow God to do so, he will add and remove exactly who he needs to from your life. Freedom from defeat and the concern of pleasing others will change your life. What pleases God? Eating healthy, speaking words of victory and living a healthy life? Or overindulging in food and drink on a regular basis even though you know it's hurting you, speaking gossip and negative words to others even though you know it will hurt someone in the end, and living a schedule that makes everyone else happy but defeats you in the meantime? Which one pleases God? The first.

Stop giving in to the people who are WITH you in life and start giving your time and attention to the ones who are FOR you. Who cares if it's only three people? I would rather have three than twenty just riding along with me defeating me with their words and trying to steer me off track from living my dreams. If God is for you, then who dare be against you? Freedom comes with forgiveness and the release of toxic thoughts and feelings. Remove it from your world. Seek forgiveness and then digest the beautiful life you're left with to live.

Make today the day you decide you will live your dreams, NO matter what the people WITH you are telling you to eat, drink or do with your life. Spend your time with the people who are FOR you. Most importantly, spend your time pleasing God and all of the rest will fall into place. Plan for peace, because it will come to you no matter what trial hits you.

SAMPLE MENU

BREAKFAST
Cinnamon Vanilla Egg White Pancake
1 tbsp cinnamon vanilla flavored almond butter
8 strawberries sliced and spread over the top

MID-MORNING SNACK
1 Vanilla apricot No Bake Protein Bar

LUNCH
4 oz Lemon Tilapia
2 cups Roasted Broccoli
3 tbsp Quinoa on top of broccoli

MID-AFTERNOON SNACK
1 scoop chocolate Jay Robb egg white protein mixed with
1 cup almond milk and
1 tbsp chocolate raspberry flax oil

DINNER
4 oz grilled bison or beef filet seasoned with Debbie's Seasoning
Large salad with Spinach and field greens, cucumber, red onion, red pepper, artichoke, pepperoncini

Salad Dressing: olive oil, apple cider vinegar, oregano, garlic, pepper, onion powder, lemon juice

DEBBIE'S MENU

5AM
6 organic egg whites into an omelet
1 cup baked green beans
8 strawberries

8AM
4 oz Bison Crock Pot Sirloin Steak with Schultz Hot Sauce on top
1 cup Spaghetti Squash
1 cup steamed green beans

11 AM
5 oz grilled chicken breast with Debbie's Seasoning and Schultz Hot Sauce on top
1 cup Spaghetti Squash
1 cup steamed green beans

2PM
6 egg white omelet
1 cup baked green beans
1 cup Spaghetti Squash
8 strawberries

5PM
5 oz grilled chicken breast with Debbie's Seasoning and Schultz Hot Sauce on Top
2 1/2 cup Spaghetti Squash
1/2 cup sautéed leeks

BILL'S HEART HEALTHY MENU

BREAKFAST
3 egg whites scrambled
3/4 scoop chocolate Jay Robb egg white protein
1/2 banana
1/4 cup steel cut Irish oats

MID-MORNING SNACK
15 walnuts

LUNCH
6 oz BBQ Shredded Chicken
1 cup mashed cauliflower
3/4 cup mashed sweet potato
6 roasted baby carrots

AFTERNOON SNACK
1 Cinnamon Roll Larabar

DINNER
6 oz Agave Salmon
2 cups Roasted Broccoli
2 tbsp brown rice sprinkled on top of broccoli
6 roasted baby carrots

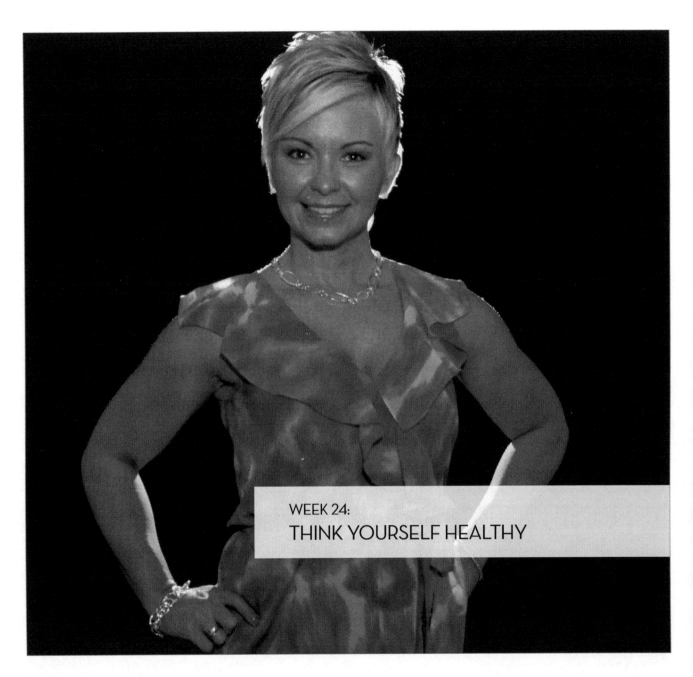

WEEK 24:
THINK YOURSELF HEALTHY

"The sum of your thoughts comprises your overall attitude." John Maxwell

What are your thoughts? Do you think you are healthy or have you accepted second best for your body, your mind and your spirit? Do you see yourself as healthy? If the sum of your thoughts comprises your attitude then I hope you think of yourself as healthy.

Don't make excuses for poor choices and continual bad decisions. If you want and need to lose weight then start seeing yourself not only as thin but as healthy. A weight loss journey is about so much more than being thin. It's about healthy living. It's a choice to change your lifestyle, no matter what your kids, spouse, friends or coworkers are choosing you choose health for yourselves.

We need to start thinking and seeing ourselves healthy; making regular and consistent healthy choices. Waking up and choosing eggs over bacon, fruit over donuts and green tea over red bull. These choices will guide you through the first few critical hours of your day. They will help build your blood sugar which will help guide you through the remainder of your day. Each choice matters. Mid-morning when your starving, have a headache and feeling and thinking your way into a bad day just think back on what your choices were for breakfast. Each meal needs to be comprised of a healthy preservative-free protein source, a clean fat source and a low glycemic unprocessed carb source. The carb source starts the fire and produces the flame and gives you that immediate energy source. Clean carb sources are fruits, vegetables and limited grains such as Ezekiel bread, quinoa, oats or brown rice. Your fat source such as the oil you use when you cook or the nuts you top your fruit with will pad the fall your body experiences when it has the carb. As you start to come down from the carb you will rest on the conserved energy of the olive oil, coconut oil, flaxseed oil or almonds or walnuts you had. Finally, as you start to fall off from your fat your body finally rests upon that healthy protein source you took in, a clean whole food source such as organic eggs, chicken, bison, turkey or salmon. Your protein is your foundation that kept your temple from falling. Each meal should hold you for approximately 3 hours. I wouldn't go much over this. Then it's time to start it all over again. Have another meal full of these choices.

When they tally up my thoughts in heaven I hope they say my thoughts of the Lord and his goodness were enormous. God is so good. He has given you this body. It is your temple. Treat it right. When you disrespect your body you are disrespecting the Lord. Choose to see yourself healthy today and make the necessary changes and CHOICES to live a health filled life.

SAMPLE MENU

BREAKFAST
Cinnamon Vanilla Egg White Pancake
1 tbsp cinnamon vanilla flavored
almond butter
8 strawberries sliced and spread
over the top

MID-MORNING SNACK
1 Vanilla apricot No Bake Protein Bar

LUNCH
Lemon Tilapia
2 cups Roasted Broccoli
3 tbsp Quinoa on top of broccoli

MID-AFTERNOON SNACK
1 scoop chocolate Jay Robb egg
white protein mixed with
1 cup almond milk and
1 tbsp chocolate raspberry flax oil

DINNER
4 oz Grilled Bison Filet of Beef
seasoned with Debbie's Seasoning
Large salad with Spinach and field
greens, cucumber, red onion, red
pepper, artichoke, pepperoncini

Salad Dressing: olive oil, apple cider
vinegar, oregano, garlic, pepper,
onion powder, lemon juice

DEBBIE'S MENU

5AM
6 organic egg whites omelet
1 cup baked green beans
8 strawberries

8AM
4 oz Bison Crock Pot Sirloin Steak
with Schultz Hot Sauce on top
1 cup Spaghetti Squash
1 cup steamed green beans

11 AM
5 oz grilled chicken breast
with Debbie's Seasoning
and Schultz Hot Sauce on top
1 cup Spaghetti Squash
1 cup steamed green beans

2PM
6 egg white omelet
1 cup baked green beans
1 cup Spaghetti Squash
8 strawberries

5PM
5 oz grilled chicken breast
with Debbie's Seasoning
and Schultz Hot Sauce on Top
2 1/2 cup Spaghetti Squash
1/2 cup sautéed leeks

BILL'S HEART HEALTHY MENU

BREAKFAST
3 egg whites, scrambled
3/4 scoop chocolate Jay Robb egg
white protein
1/2 banana
1/4 cup steel cut Irish oats

MID-MORNING SNACK
15 walnuts

LUNCH
6 oz BBQ Shredded Chicken
1 cup mashed cauliflower
3/4 cup mashed sweet potato
6 roasted baby carrots

AFTERNOON SNACK
1 Cinnamon Roll Larabar

DINNER
6 oz Agave Salmon
2 cups Roasted Broccoli
2 tbsp brown rice sprinkled on
top of broccoli
6 roasted baby carrots

ARTIFICIAL SWEETENERS: WHAT YOU DON'T KNOW CAN HURT YOU

Artificial sweeteners were designed to be sugar substitutes as a less fattening alternative. These sugar substitutes are virtually ubiquitous and mimic the flavor of sugar, but with virtually no useful energy.

Aspartame is a non-saccharine artificial sweetener currently used in over 6,000 diet and low-calorie food products. Popular trademark brands of the sweetener in the United States include NutraSweet®, Equal®, and Tropicana Slim®. There are thousands of everyday products that contain aspartame including, yogurt, sodas, pudding, tabletop sugar substitutes, and chewing gum. Research done on aspartame has shown that it may not be completely safe for human consumption and may cause a number of health complications if taken in large doses. Efforts to revoke FDA approval on aspartame have been unsuccessful, so it is advisable to simply avoid these products whenever possible.

Aspartame is made up of three chemicals: aspartic acid, phenylalanine, and methanol. The ingestion of excess aspartic acid from aspartame and other excess free excitatory amino acids can cause serious chronic neurological disorders and a myriad of other acute symptoms. Aspartic acid is an amino acid. Taken in its free form, it significantly raises the blood plasma level of aspartate and glutamate. Aspartate and glutamate act as excitatory neurotransmitters in the brain by facilitating synaptic transmission, which triggers excessive amounts of free radicals, killing the cells. The large majority of neural cells in a particular area of the brain are killed before any clinical symptoms of a chronic illness are noticed. Aspartame is an NMDA receptor antagonist, which means that it inhibits the release of neurotransmitters that cause pain within the body.

Studies report a range of side-effects including fibromyalgia, brain tumors, mental retardation, birth defects, epilepsy, memory loss, lymphoma, leukemia, diabetes, Parkinson's disease, and peripheral nerve cancer. Headaches and migraine symptoms are one of the most common side effects of aspartame.

Splenda, aka sucralose, is a synthetic compound stumbled upon in 1976 by scientists in Britain seeking a new pesticide formulation. It is another alternative sweetener currently on the market, often labeled as "Reduced Sugar" products. Products featuring Splenda are perceived as "natural" because the FDA's press release about sucralose parrots the claim that "it is made from sugar." At least 15% of ingested Splenda is not excreted by the kidneys. It seems to sequester in the nervous system, gut, sensory apparatuses, muscles or in the circulatory systems. The severity of adverse reactions varies genetically. Scientists are calling Splenda a mild mutagen, based on how much is absorbed.

Typical reactions from Splenda ingestion occur immediately or up to eleven hours after ingestion and affect nearly every physiological system in the body, including the nervous system and brain, gastrointestinal tract, epidermis, electrical conduction of the heart and cardiovascular system, sensory receptors, musculoskeletal system, and the genitourinary tract.

Food additives—including artificial sweeteners—are not subject to the same gauntlet of FDA safety trials as pharmaceuticals. In addition, most of the testing is funded by the food industry, which has a vested interest in the outcome.

ALTERNATIVES TO ARTIFICIAL SWEETENERS: THE NATURAL WAY

Agave, as compared to other sweeteners, has a desirable low-glycemic index. This means that when consumed, it won't cause a sharp rise or fall in blood sugar. Agave contains saponins and fructans. Saponins have anti-inflammatory and immune system-boosting properties, including antimicrobial capability. Inulin is a type of fructan that has many health benefits. Studies suggest that inulin can be effective in weight loss because of its low impact on blood sugar and its ability to increase satiety and decrease appetite. Inulin is also associated with lowering cholesterol, reducing the risk of certain cancers, and increasing the absorption of nutrients, such as isoflavones, calcium and magnesium. In addition, fructans are not destroyed in the stomach and may be a delivery system for drugs to treat colon diseases.

Stevia serves as a remarkable natural sweetener. Stevia is a small shrub that is 300 to 400 times sweeter than regular sugar. It contains no calories and is nutritious as well as non-toxic. Scientific research has indicated that it regulates blood sugar, lowers blood pressure, inhibits the growth and reproduction of bacteria and infectious organisms, reduces cravings for sweet and fatty foods, regulates the hypothalamic hunger mechanism, and improves gastrointestinal function.

Xylitol is a naturally occurring carbohydrate. It is found in fibrous vegetables and fruit, and is produced metabolically. Pure xylitol is a white crystalline substance that looks and tastes like sugar. While xylitol is just as sweet as table sugar (sucrose), it has about 40% fewer calories and 75% fewer carbohydrates. Importantly, xylitol is slowly absorbed and metabolized, resulting in very negligible changes in insulin. Xylitol therefore won't raise blood sugar like regular sugar, which places tremendous strain on your system, causing negative health effects.

ALTERNATIVES TO DIET SODA AND ENERGY DRINKS

Energy drinks and diet sodas have become the two fastest selling categories in the beverage industry. What gives these drinks their kick? There are no secret ingredients here. Caffeine, sugar, and artificial sweeteners are abundant throughout the beverage industry.

Artificial sweeteners are marketed with the promise of weight control, and the blind acceptance of these, such as sucralose (aka Splenda) and aspartame (aka Nutrasweet), plays a significant role in the massive array of health issues that plague society today. Seeing as diet soda and energy drinks are among the most popular beverages on the market, it may seem nearly impossible to avoid these drinks altogether. The havoc these toxins wreak on overall health is a large price to pay for a simple "caffeine fix" or to "kill a craving." Several healthy, alternative options are listed below that will not wreak havoc on hormones, electrolyte balance, energy and mood levels, or neurotransmitter conduction and reception.

CocoPure: CocoPure is a concentrated cocoa tea blend, bursting with 4,000 mg of concentrated cocoa that offers a powerhouse of antioxidant protection against free radical damage. In addition, the health-giving benefits of CocoPure have been further increased by adding green tea and resveratrol. This unique combination of ingredients supports cardiovascular health, arterial health, increased blood flow, digestive health,

immune system support, and healthy energy levels. CocoPure is great as a drink by itself mixed with hot water or mixed into other items, such as coffee, protein shakes, unsweetened almond or coconut milk, oatmeal, yogurt, and much more!

Coffee/Espresso: While brewing beverages at home is always the best option because it allows for complete control over what goes into the drink, there are a few options at your local coffee shop that fit easily into a clean eating and healthy lifestyle. Espresso and coffee alone are virtually calorie-free. A cup of black coffee contains a mere 5 calories and espresso has a mere 10 calories. When ordering, always ask the server to leave room in the cup (should you prefer to add your own almond milk or Stevia) and order beverages plain. The table below provides a comparison of self-sweetened beverages versus staff-sweetened.

To achieve the coffee shop taste without paying the heavy caloric prices, sweeten beverages with unsweetened almond milk or coconut milk. To spice things up, add additional sweeteners and spices

DRINK THIS, NOT THAT	
YES	Healthy Caffé Latte- 35 calories, 1.5g fat, 1g carbs, 1g protein
NO	Caffé Latte- 190 calories, 7g fat, 18g carbs, 12g protein
YES	Healthy Caffé Mocha- 55 calories, 1.5g fat, 1g carbs, 1g protein
NO	Caffé Mocha- 260 calories, 8g fat, 41g carbs, 13g protein
YES	Healthy Caramel Macchiato- 35 calories, 1.5g fat, 1g carbs, 1g protein
NO	Caramel Macchiato- 240 calories, 7g fat, 34g carbs, 10g protein
YES	Healthy Cinnamon Dolce Latte- 40 calories, 1.5g fat,1g carbs, 1g protein
NO	Cinnamon Dolce Latte- 260 calories, 6g fat, 40g carbs, 11g protein
YES	Healthy Vanilla Latte- 35 calories, 1.5g fat, 1g carbs, 1g protein
NO	Vanilla Latte- 250 calories, 6g fat, 36g carbs, 12g protein
YES	Healthy Pumpkin Spice Latte- 40 calories, 1.5g fat, 1g carbs, 1g protein
NO	Pumpkin Spice Latte- 310 calories, 6g fat, 49g carbs, 14g protein

** All nutritional information is from www.starbucks.com and includes a grande (16oz) beverage with 2% milk and regular sweeteners.

to taste such as cinnamon, alcohol-free vanilla extract, pumpkin pie spice, agave, and Stevia (which comes in a variety of liquid flavors, such as vanilla, chocolate, toffee, caramel, and more).

Tea: Several varieties of tea have an equivalent amount of caffeine to provide a quick burst of energy. Many coffee shops also brew teas, served hot or cold, and are all calorie-free. Ordering options include: Tazo® Awake Tea, Tazo® Green Tea, Tazo® Earl Grey Tea, Tazo® Orange Blossom Tea, Tazo® Passion Tea, Tazo® Vanilla Rooibos Tea, etc. All teas can be sweetened with Stevia as needed or made into a latte with the addition of unsweetened almond milk or coconut milk. Local grocery stores offer a variety of fair-trade certified organic teas that can easily be brewed at home. Popular brands include Yogi Tea, Revolution Tea, Celestial Seasonings, Choice Tea, Organic Tea, and much more!

THE TRUTH ABOUT FRUIT: THE MYTH ABOUT FRUIT AND FITNESS

The phrase "An apple a day keeps the doctor away" may no longer be a valid statement. Glucose and fructose, simple carbohydrates utilized for basic metabolic processes in the body, may have similar chemical structures, but this does not necessarily mean they are processed in the same manner. In fact, there is much speculation about the physiological variances between glucose and fructose metabolism. A recent study examined the effects of glucose, fructose, and normal saline (as a control) on hypothalamic function. According to The Chicago Tribune, "glucose significantly raised levels of neural activity for 20 minutes following the infusion. Fructose had the opposite effect, causing activities…to drop and stay low for 20 minutes after the infusion." This has a significant effect on the American population because fructose, in the form of high-fructose corn syrup, is now a staple ingredient in all types of foods. From canned soups to boxed cereals, baked goods to frozen meats, condiments to sodas, high-fructose corn syrup remains abundant and the number one source of calories in Americans. While only time will tell what the more defined results of this study entail, it is clear that fructose is detrimental to an area of the brain involved in hormone production and appetite control.

What makes fructose different from any other sugar? Fructose is entirely metabolized by the liver, which means that excess fructose is not only harmful to the liver, but is also converted to adipose fat. This type of fat deposits around the abdomen and leads to other comorbidities, such as obesity, hypertension, diabetes, and dyslipidemia, all of which are significant risk factors for cardiovascular disease according to the ACC/AHA guidelines. Glucose is the primary source of energy for metabolic processes and excess fructose will merely be stored as fat. In addition, fructose has no suppressive effect on ghrelin and leptin, hormones that stimulate appetite. As a result, overeating occurs due to the lack of negative feedback inhibition on hypothalamic synthesis and release of these hormones. What makes high-fructose corn syrup even worse? High-fructose corn syrup is about 55% fructose; in its liquid form, its negative metabolic effects increase dramatically. Furthermore, high-fructose corn syrup is often synthesized from genetically modified corn, laden with its own host of adverse effects and health concerns.

Naturally occurring fructose is bonded to a myriad of other sugars, decreasing its metabolic toxicity.

Table sugar (aka sucrose), is a 1:1 ratio of fructose to glucose, meaning its molecular structure is comprised of 50% fructose molecules and 50% glucose molecules. Based upon previous statements, it appears as if table sugar is the healthier option. However, this is not the case. While glucose in itself does not cause insulin resistance, it does increase absorption of fructose when ingested simultaneously. This being said, if cane sugar is naturally extracted from the plant and not synthetically compounded in a factory, it is still only marginally healthier.

Upon ingestion, 100% of fructose is absorbed from the intestine and transported via the portal vein to the liver. There, it undergoes a series of reactions to form two different intermediates that lead to increased fat deposition. Fructose-1,6-bisphosphate can be converted to dihydroxyacetone-phosphate which functions in fatty acid esterification (synthesis of triglycerides). The other compound, glyceradehyde-3-phosphate is directly converted to free fatty acids. Despite the fact these compounds will get stored, fructose also provides the necessary components to increase hepatic production of

VLDL (damaging cholesterol), the precursor to LDL (bad cholesterol). The free fatty acids that are not utilized for metabolic purposes accumulate as droplets in the liver and skeletal muscle tissues, leading to insulin resistance (and ultimately Type II Diabetes Mellitus) and Non-alcoholic Fatty Liver Disease. The metabolism of fructose in the liver results in a myriad of toxic by products. A prominent byproduct is uric acid, a compound that may increase blood pressure and cause or worsen gout.

All in all, it is essential to understand that dietary fat alone does not lead to obesity, but excess carbohydrates, fructose in particular, play a significant role. As a standard recommendation, limit total consumption of fructose to 15-20g daily. This will require limiting hidden sources of fructose, including condiments, beverages, and processed food. Be sure to check the label on all products and beware of sugar in any form (molasses, honey, agave, sugar, etc) and any ingredient that ends in –ose, as this indicates a type of carbohydrate. To the right is a reference table with common fruits and the amount of fructose in each.

FRUIT	SERVING SIZE	G/FRUCTOSE
Limes	1 medium	0
Lemons	1 medium	0.6
Cranberries	1 cup	0.7
Passion fruit	1 medium	0.9
Prune	1 medium	1.2
Apricot	1 medium	1.3
Guava	1 medium	2.2
Date (Deglet Noor)	2 medium	2.6
Cantaloupe	1/8 medium melon	2.8
Raspberries	1 cup	3.0
Clementine	1 medium	3.4
Kiwifruit	1 medium	3.4
Blackberries	1 cup	3.5
Starfruit	1 medium	3.6
Cherries, sweet	10	3.8
Strawberries	1 cup	3.8
Cherries, sour	1 cup	4.0
Pineapple	1 slice (3.5" x 0.75")	4.0
Grapefruit	1/2 medium	4.3
Boysenberries	1 cup	4.6
Tangerine	1 medium	4.8
Nectarine	1 medium	5.4
Peach	1 medium	5.9
Orange (navel)	1 medium	6.1
Papaya	1/2 medium	6.3
Honeydew	1/8 medium melon	6.7
Banana	1 medium	7.1
Blueberries	1 cup	7.4
Date (Meejol)	1 medium	7.7
Apple	1 medium	9.5
Persimmon	1 medium	10.6
Watermelon	1/16 medium melon	11.3
Pear	1 medium	11.8
Raisins	1/4 cup	12.3
Grapes	1 cup	12.4
Mango	1/2 medium	16.2
Apricots, dried	1 cup	16.4
Figs, dried	1 cup	23.0

FALSE HEALTH CLAIMS: THE TRUTH ABOUT SOY

Soy is NOT the acclaimed health food as advertised today. Soy products have swept the nation as a natural, healthy alternative source of protein. However, new studies raise questions over whether the ingredients in soy might increase the risk of breast cancer in some women, affect brain function in men and lead to hidden developmental abnormalities in infants.

The core of concerns rests with the chemical makeup of soy: in addition to all the nutrients and protein, soy contains a natural chemical that mimics estrogen, the female hormone. Studies show this alters development; in fact, two glasses of soy milk per day over the course of one month contain enough of the chemical to change the timing of a woman's menstrual cycle.

Soybeans contain an impressive array of phytochemicals (biologically active components derived from plants), the most interesting of which are known as isoflavones. Isoflavones are the compounds which are being studied in relation to the relief of certain menopausal symptoms, cancer prevention, slowing or reversing osteoporosis and reducing the risk of heart disease. Unfortunately soybeans, as provided by nature, are not suitable for human consumption. Only after fermentation for some time, or extensive processing, including chemical extractions and high temperatures, is the soy protein isolate, suitable for digestion when eaten. Soybeans also reportedly contain the highest level of an anti-nutrient called "phytic acid," which may block the absorption of certain minerals including magnesium, calcium, iron and zinc. Adding to the high phytate problem, soybeans are highly resistant to phytate-reducing techniques, such as long, slow cooking. Soybeans contain potent enzyme-inhibitors that block uptake of trypsin and other enzymes needed by the body for protein digestion. Normal cooking does not deactivate these harmful antinutrients, which can cause serious gastric distress, reduced protein digestion and can lead to chronic deficiencies in amino acid uptake. In addition, soybeans also contain hemagglutinin, a clot-promoting substance which causes red blood cells to clump together. These clustered blood cells cannot properly absorb oxygen for distribution to the body's tissues and are unable to help in maintaining good cardiac health. Hemagglutinin and trypsin inhibitors are both "growth depressant" substances. Although the act of fermenting soybeans does deactivate both hemagglutinin and trypsin inhibitors, cooking and precipitation do not. Although these enzyme inhibitors are found in reduced levels within precipitated soy products like tofu, they are not completely eliminated.

Over 90% of soy is genetically modified and has one of the highest contamination percentages by pesticides compared to all other foods. Soy processors have worked hard to get these anti-nutrients out of the finished product, particularly soy protein isolate, which is the key ingredient in most soy foods. Production takes place in industrial factories where soybeans are first mixed with an alkaline solution to remove fiber, then precipitated and separated using an acid wash and finally, neutralized in an alkaline solution. Acid washing in aluminum tanks leaches high levels of aluminum into the final product. As a result, soy-based products may contain up to 1000% more aluminum. The milk protein is hydrolyzed 80%, which tends to significantly decrease its tendency to cause allergic reactions. Finally, the resulting products are spray-dried at high temperatures to produce a high-protein powder. A final hardship to the original soybean is high-temperature, high-pressure extrusion processing of soy protein isolate to produce textured vegetable protein. Nitrites, potent carcinogens, are formed during spray-drying and a toxin called "lysinoalanine" is formed during alkaline processing.

All in all, soy consumption should be completely eliminated due to the extensive array of adverse effects and high chemical processing during production. The minimal health benefits of soy are completely overshadowed by its large potential for health destruction.

TESTIMONIALS

BILL CLARK, FATHER

This book will change how you look at the food you eat. You can eat a lot and still maintain your weight, feel good and maintain your energy. I don't get tired or hungry.
In August 2010 I suffered a heart attack. I was unconscious for 14 days and went through a quadruple bypass heart operation. When leaving the hospital I started a diet plan designed for me by Debbie from foods and recipes identified in this book. With her support, my wife Barb and Deb's sister and brother, Kim and Bob, I have continued to grow and improve for the past year of recovery.

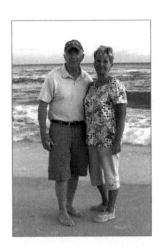

The food has been great. Everything tastes great! There is no getting bored with eating the same plain thing every day. You have a lot of choices that others don't provide to you. I have gone through cardiac rehab and the dieting information they have provided has been disappointing. I do continue the rehab exercise program along with Debbie's food. Three days a week doing 40 minutes cardio and about 30 minutes light weights.

The last year I have maintained my weight not varying more than one pound. The most my weight ever changed was one pound.

It is easier to prevent than it is to recover.
Read this book and enjoy your life!

BRITTANY BEGGS

In today's society, it's not easy keeping up with the best eating habits, but practicing better eating habits, in time becomes instinctive. About seven years ago, while I was studying in college, I noticed my waistline kept growing each year. I didn't eat large quantities, in fact, I didn't really eat much at all, maybe 1-2 meals a day. Watching my waistline grow, I knew I had to do something. That year, I started weight training. I saw gradual progress, but nothing significant. It wasn't until six years later, with school almost finished, that I decided it was time to take care of myself. I started eating clean and training hard in January 2011. In the short period of three weeks, I saw results. My clothes fit looser, and friends and family started to notice too. Not only was I able to see my body change, and look the best it ever has, I was able to learn how to eat clean and learn what my body likes and dislikes. Every body is different, and experimenting I learned, is important.

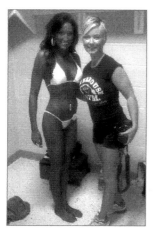

These small changes, soon became exponential. I learned, that as I took better care of myself, the quality of my life improved. I've grown tremendously in this short time, physically, mentally, and spiritually and I'm excited to continue this journey. I was only given one body, and I must take care of it!

FRANCINE VOSS

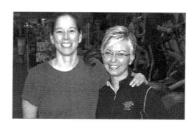

Debbie has been my personal trainer for about one year now, and the experience has been life changing for me.

Last year, and every year prior, I worked out every day, thought that I was eating right, but wasn't getting results that I wanted. I hired Debbie after noticing how effective she was with other clients. Debbie not only provided routines that took each individual to their personal limit, she gave nutritional advice, and a constant stream of encouragement.

After training with Debbie, I've altered my diet, my workouts, and cardio. I haven't lost any weight, but my family and co-workers keep asking me if I have. My husband has also noticed a difference in my body and tells me that I'm shapely.

The most significant change was one that I didn't anticipate, My weekly migraines have ceased. I could count on the headache starting Thursday afternoon, get progressively worse on Friday, and keep me on the couch with the shades pulled on Saturday. I'd start to recover on Sunday, only to repeat the process next week. To put this in perspective, that equates to approximately 156 days of headache.

However, the headaches are now gone and I'm certain that it is a result of a diet that is right for me, coupled with the intense workout. I can enjoy Saturdays with my husband Phil again, and give my best at work during the week. As I mentioned before – it's life changing. I can't thank Debbie enough for providing expertise, motivation and encouragement every week!

KRISTEN CRAWFORD

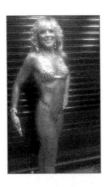

My experience at Powerhouse Gym and working with Debbie has been exceptionally fulfilling and motivating. As a competitive gymnast throughout my childhood, I have always been driven and competitive. However, I struggled to find a sport I could compete in successfully at this age and stage in my life. Debbie introduced me to the sport of body building and figure competitions, and she has played a crucial role in helping me to achieve my nutritional and fitness goals, culminating in competing in my first body building competition at age 43! I am now as fit and lean as I was in my twenties. Through her help, I've lost 10 pounds, developed much better lean muscle mass and definition, and comfortably fit into my size 2 clothing! In addition, I have greater energy and less fatigue. As a former vegetarian, I would never have dreamed that I would look and feel better while consuming a diet much higher in protein, but she has changed my mind and helped me to adopt a new lifestyle.

Her positive energy, zest for life and passion for her work kept me going at times when it would have been easier to quit. I now look forward to achieving a level of fitness that I wouldn't have thought possible five years ago. My next short-term goal is to win a body building competition, and long-term to remain the same size and weight at age 50 as I currently am today. I am confident that I will not only achieve this, but through Debbie's help I will set and achieve new goals that I never would have had the courage to attempt.

RACHEL LANDES

It was almost four years ago that I first stepped into Powerhouse Gym. A friend had recommended I visit and see if it was right for me. I planned on competing in a pageant which included my first ever swimsuit competition. Knowing this, I realized that I had to get into the best shape of my life. I began working out twice a week with a Powerhouse Gym personal trainer and signed on to receive nutritional counseling, too. Needless to say, with the hard work, dedication, and inspiration of the Powerhouse Gym staff, my trainer, and nutritionist, I began to look and feel the best I ever had in my life.

After the first year of training, I was hooked. I continued competing and continued my training for the next three years. I've learned how to eat and work out and I've gained confidence that I truly believe comes from taking pride in a healthy body and mind.

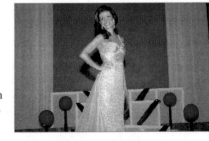

There's no better feeling than being able to crank out a set of push-ups with the best of them or keep up right alongside the boys in the gym. Working with my personal trainer and nutritionist has changed my life and helped me to become the confident and proud woman I am today. It is, without a doubt, the best decision I've ever made.

SARA BROWN

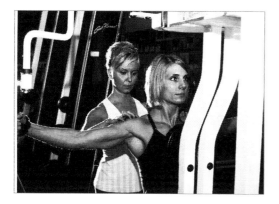

On my journey to my first figure competition I had to learn to eat clean. This required a lot of pre-planning at first, because I couldn't just pick up fast food whenever I felt hungry, or buy pre-packaged meals. Once clean eating became a habit, it was a lot easier to maintain than I expected. Now I have a shopping list when I go to the store and spend less because I'm not tempted to buy things I know my body won't utilize. I can see myself continuing to eat this way for the rest of my life because I want to be at my best physically, and I need to be healthy to do all the things I want to do. My new eating habits have started to trickle over into other areas of my life. I've begun to maximize my full potential by re-examining the big picture, getting my priorities in line with my dreams and goals. A photograph shows how I changed my outward appearance but the real change was inner. Anyone can do this. All it takes is a decision to get started!

JAMIE CREGGER

I approached Debbie at the gym and asked her if she would be able to train me before my wedding. Not only did she help me look great on my wedding day but she inspired me to make a significant lifestyle change. This lifestyle change would allow me to feel good about myself and give me the energy to fuel my busy life.

We discussed my diet in great detail. It was clear that I needed to make some changes in order to achieve my goal of looking and feeling better. Debbie gave me healthier and cleaner options to take the place of the many processed foods I was putting in my body. I slowly began to make these changes and could see and feel the impact right away. She also set up a cardio schedule of 40 minutes 4 days a week.

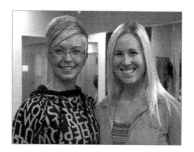

Six years later, I have kept this schedule intact. By keeping my diet clean, I have been able to maintain a healthy weight without having to kill it in the gym for hours every night.

By having a regular workout routine and keeping consistent with my clean and healthy eating, I was also able to maintain a healthy weight during pregnancy and after my son was born I was able to get back to my normal weight quickly. I honestly don't think I could have done this without Debbie.

TORI TAGGART

For almost as long as I can remember, I have had all sorts of digestive issues. I spent years of my adolescence

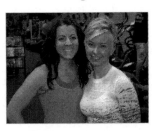

getting test, after scan, without a "real" diagnosis, being told time after time, that it was all in my head, that my problems were stress-related and was given a new medicine to try and sent on my way, always to no prevail. I sort of sloughed it off, feeling like "This is just the way I am"and will always be.

I am a very active person, spending most of my free time running or in the gym and a very healthy eater. I have always been careful about what I eat following all the "typical" rules, (even having a food allergy/sensitivity tests done) and yet I just wasn't feeling good. I was tired, fatigued, exhausted even diagnosed with "Adrenal Fatigue." My digestive issues seemed to never improve, my memory was suffering, and I could not lose a pound to save my life. Things just seemed to be getting worse and I finally decided to make an appointment with Debbie. After speaking with Debbie,

I went home with a new plan in hand. She not only gave me a nutrition plan, but she spelled it out for me, recipe by recipe and made it easy to follow. Within the first week I felt significant improvement. I even remember asking myself why I hadn't done this sooner!

AMY LESCHER

I am a 36 year old mother of two beautiful girls. I grew up very athletic, playing softball, soccer and dancing. After having my second child at 35, I found myself unmotivated and left with a bunch of baby weight that wasn't coming off very easily. I worked out on my own for a couple of months, dropped some weight, but was still searching for more. That's when I decided it's now or never…if I want to fulfill my dream of competing, there is no time like the present!

I can still remember my consult session with Deb. She identified all of my imbalances and flexibility issues and gave me simple corrective exercises to do on a daily basis as well as a foam roller program. One of my major issues was rounded shoulders, and I seriously thought I had excellent posture. However, within six weeks, no more rounded shoulders for me and I appeared an inch taller and no longer had neck tension. I still do these today!

The first training session I thought I would die! It was legs. I had never sweat so much in my life! I literally thought I needed help walking to my car and then I had to go home where my bedroom is on the second level, which was sure fun!

Over a six month period I worked with Debbie and Roger. They completely transformed me. I felt great and never had been in that kind of shape! I went from an out of shape mom to a figure competitor who had no excuses! Complete strangers would approach me at the gym and want to know how they can change.

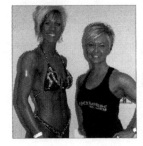

I completed in my first competition in July 2011 and finished first in two categories. I was ecstatic! I have Debbie Portell to thank immensely for helping me to achieve a lifelong dream!!

MISTY SOWELL

I am a 36 year old mother of five beautiful healthy children! And feel I am in the best shape of my life!

I started working out about nine years ago. My youngest wasn't quite a year but I remember feeling just absolutely...blah! I had no energy, completely exhausted daily and found myself laying on the couch watching my kids play rather than playing "with" them. I hated that! Too tired for the hair, makeup and regular clothes and even friends, it was sweats and a baggy t-shirt everywhere I went. It was when one of my children asked me if we could go to the park to play and I sadly answered, "Oh sweetie, Mommy's too tired right now. Maybe later." I will always remember the look on his face and the feeling in the pit of my stomach, thinking, "This is not the kind of Mother I wanted to be!" I thought, "something's wrong." So, I made an appointment with my doctor. After blood work, etc., and nothing came back abnormal, he looked at me and said "You are a Mom of five, you should be tired" I thought. "No, I just simply wasn't going to accept that." Well, I joined a gym.

Four years ago a lady from out of town came in to the gym one night and was just stacked with muscle! I wanted that! I got up the nerve to ask her what she does. She said she used to meet with a nutritionist in Missouri, his name is Roger. I got the number, called him the next day, and well, like they say the rest is history! I never saw her again actually. It's weird but amazing how people come into your life. This man is one of the most knowledgeable men I know. I learned how to eat, the first key to success in your weight loss goals. After working with Roger for about a year, I started working out with Debbie Portell and set a goal to compete!! Yes, a mom of five competing! On stage in that little bikini! How grateful and truly blessed I am to have Debbie and Roger in my life. I wouldn't be where I am today if it wasn't for those two! They have come into my life and shown me how to live a healthy and active lifestyle. After having five kids I am truly in the best shape my life! And most importantly I have the energy to play with my kids! And to me, that is everything! I now look forward to going to the gym six times a week and sharing that passion with others! I am a certified personal trainer and a Zumba Instructor. I also am looking forward to competing in my 3rd figure competition in June. If I can do it, you can do it! I can't tell you it's easy, I can only tell you it's worth it! Where there's a will there's a way! And trust me, we can come up with an excuse pretty easily to not make it into the gym. Laundry, meals to make, grocery shopping, bathrooms, more laundry, bathing kids, homework, driving kids to and from sports or dance and the list goes on...but I truly believe, we are ALL STRONGER than excuses!

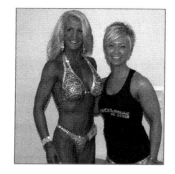

LIBBY HERMAN

My experience with nutrition and training is a never-ending process, as I am always open to new ideas and willing to listen to those who teach. I had very limited knowledge when I joined Powerhouse Gym. As an 85 pound anorexic girl, I thought I knew all there was to know about dieting. After all, I read every fitness magazine on the shelf, spent countless hours researching various approaches to dieting, and looked up just about every reduced calorie recipe on the planet. But, when I finally realized I was unhealthy, I couldn't seem to budge the scale past the 90 pound mark. I did not understand why I wasn't seeing progress. After all, I was consuming more calories than before!

After faltering somewhere between the 90 and 95 pound mark, I decided it was time to take matters out of my own hands. A friend advised me to talk to Roger, the owner of Powerhouse Gym, as he is very well renowned in the fitness industry and incredibly knowledgeable. I sent Roger an e-mail, and he responded immediately, offering me a free orientation. Nervous, I entered his office, anxious to hear his advice and apprehensive at the thought of what he would recommend. Admittedly, I was intimidated, but Roger was very professional. He outlined every single meal in precise detail and explained the purpose of each nutrient at the specific times of day. I could not have asked for more. Being an anorexic, I was accustomed to having every detail of my meals planned.

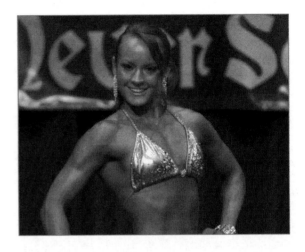

Afterwards, Roger introduced me to Debbie, initially just to copy down her meatloaf recipe. However, after discovering I was interested in competing in a figure competition, Debbie and Roger led me through a fitness orientation. Flabbergasted, I could not believe I had so many muscular imbalances and was not maximizing my workouts to their full potential! It was simply unbelievable. I immediately began training with Debbie twice weekly from that moment on. Workouts with Debbie were challenging, to say the least. After each session, not only was I exhausted, but I was astounded at how much weight I was able to lift or how hard I was able to push myself. My second workout with her was a leg day; I literally thought I was going to die. I made it out alive, albeit barely, and experienced difficulty walking and/or sitting for the next week. Workouts definitely progressed as my body adapted to the intense workload. Even more amazing than the fact she was able to push me through seemingly insurmountable workouts, was her incessant and vast knowledge of training and nutrition. Reasons for each exercise, explanations of the specific order of exercises, descriptions on how each movement operates within the body, depictions of exact proper alignment during each movement (down to the toe position), and clarifications on how each exercise would affect my muscular imbalances streamed endlessly from Debbie's lips, as I listened each and every session, hoping to absorb a fraction of her knowledge. I left each session feeling exhausted, enlightened, and uplifted.

Despite all of my struggles through school, work, life, and training, Debbie always maintained a positive attitude for me and all of her clients. She lifts my spirits whenever I am depressed and always has faith in me. I cannot think of a more perfect trainer. Admirable, kind, generous, honest, intelligent, and faithful are only a few of the adjectives to describe her personality. Her unique approach to training and everlasting positivity astound me. She truly is a one-of-a-kind, role model.

With Roger's vast knowledge of nutrition and Debbie's unprecedented knowledge of training, I watched my body transform from skin and bone to lean muscle in no time. Just three short months later, I weighed 125lbs and was about 14 percent body fat. I absolutely love my physique and was simply speechless. I continued to work with Debbie and Roger as they guided me through my first figure competition, where I placed fifth. This was quite an accomplishment, as my path to health and fitness was quite different from others; not to mention, I was the youngest competitor on stage and had only been seriously lifting for approximately ten months. The two worked seamlessly in tandem, one complementing the other. The intricate workings of both Debbie and Roger had synergistic effects that propelled my physique in an un-paralleled fashion. Each one knew how to make minor adjustments and worked cooperatively to achieve the best results. It was a truly wonderful experience and I could not have hoped for more.

Throughout my diet and training for my competition, as well as for a significant period afterward, Roger worked endlessly to attempt to fix my gastrointestinal issues. I met with him almost daily to update him on how my body responded to certain foods, and he would adjust as needed. He recommended doctors and explained the exact details of each regimen. Most importantly, Roger and Debbie both cared for my overall health. No matter how bizarre a certain food regimen seemed, Roger would explain the scientific and physiological basis for each. When all else failed, he continued to research and implement new dietary regimens. My health improved daily, as did my knowledge and appreciation for the nutritional value of food.

Debbie never ceased caring for me. Not only did she continue to supplement Roger's dietary knowledge, she expanded my training knowledge past what I thought was possible. Never once did I feel as if a workout was sub-par. We rarely performed the same exercises twice. She always listened to my requests and incorporated them into future workouts. Each workout with Debbie was the highlight of my day. I genuinely looked forward to getting to spend those sacred 52 minutes with her, even if most of them were spent breathless and in pain. Words of encouragement and never defeat always came from Debbie's mouth. Not once did I hear her complain, gossip, or utter a single word of negativity. She remains, to this day, the light at the end of a dark tunnel for me. I trust that I can always seek her advice and never fear judgment, ridicule, or chastisement.

Both Debbie and Roger showed me extraordinary care and passion. My training and nutrition experience with the two of them was absolutely incredible. To this day, I hope to be half of the beautiful person that Debbie is and retain half

of Roger's knowledge. I am truly honored to have experienced such a wonderfully unique, compassionate, dedicated, and knowledgeable program such as that formulated by Roger and Debbie. The changes they have instilled in me will remain with me forever, as will their caring generosity and loving kindness.

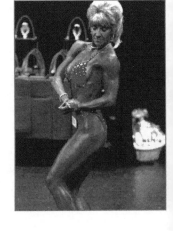

CINDY MANTIA

After reaching my heaviest weight of 196 pounds., I worked out on my own for several months with minimal results. I then hired a personal trainer and nutrition coach and learned how to work out and eat the correct way. Eighteen months later I competed for the first time in a bodybuilding and figure show weighing in at 126 pounds. I took first in Masters Figure and received my Pro Card. In the same evening I also won first in Sub-Masters and second in Novice Bodybuilding. I can't thank Debbie enough for helping me achieve such great results. With her help I have committed to living a healthy lifestyle. With clean eating and exercising, my life has become much more rewarding. To this day she is still my trainer, Thank you Debbie.

RECIPES

MEATS

Sloppy Joes
Grass Fed Meatloaf
Melt in your Mouth Roast
Agave Chili Sauce Bison Burger
Bison Beef Stew
BBQ Bison Meatloaf
Bison Chili
Bison Crock Pot Sirloin
Bison Flank Steak
BBQ Bison Roast
Bison Roast
Grilled Bison Sirloin Steak
French Onion Bison Beef Tips
Hulkburger
Roasted Bison Flank Steak
Shredded BBQ Bison Roast
Spicy Bison Stew

FISH

Agave Grilled Salmon
Baked Balsamic Pineapple Salmon
Baked Cod
Baked Lemon Garlic Salmon
Cranberry Pineapple Salmon
Crunchy Lemon-Pepper
    Grilled Salmon
Mustard Encrusted Tilapia
Lemon Garlic Tilapia
Pan-Seared Ezekiel Bread Crumb
    Encrusted Tilapia
Pan-Seared Tilapia
Pan-Seared Tuna Steak Salad
Roasted Salmon and
    Asparagus Salad

Salmon Salad
Seasoned Tilapia
Tilapia Salad

POULTRY

Chicken Chili
Debbie's Seasoned Chicken
Chicken Fingers
Crunchy Chicken Dijon
Ezekiel Bread Crumb Encrusted
    Chicken Cutlet
Grilled Chicken Wing Cutlets
Hot Chicken Salad
Lemon Chicken
Lemon-Garlic Roasted
    Turkey Breast
Pan-Seared Chicken
Roasted BBQ Chicken
Shredded BBQ Chicken
BBQ Chicken
Spicy Chicken Wingettes
Spicy Orange Chicken
Grain-Free Turkey Meatloaf
Turkey Meatloaf
Whole Oven-Baked Chicken

VEGGIES

Baked Green Beans
Baked Sweet Potatoes
Baked Sweet Potato Fries
Caramelized Balsamic Onions
Chow Chow
Cole Slaw
Crisp Citrus Salad
Grapefruit Salad

Kale Chips
Lemon Pepper Roasted Broccoli
Mashed Cauliflower
Mashed Sweet Potato
Roasted Asparagus
Roasted Balsamic Asparagus
Roasted Broccoli
Roasted Broccoli with Garlic
Roasted Carrots
Roasted Red Peppers
Roasted Red Pepper and
    Red Onion
Roasted Tomatoes
Roasted Zucchini
Spaghetti Squash

BREAKFAST

Apple Cinnamon Pancake
Blueberry Banana Pancake
Cinnamon Vanilla Egg
    White Pancake
Egg White French Toast
Equal Parts Pancake
Pumpkin Pancake
Sweet Potato Pancake
Zucchini Pancake

SNACKS

Chocolate P.Nut Butter Bar
Cinnamon Vanilla Trail Mix
Original Protein Bar
Strawberry Protein Bar
Vanilla Apricot Protein Bar
Pumpkin Protein Bar

MEATS

BEEF

Sloppy Joes

1 lb organic grass fed lean ground sirloin

1 can organic tomato sauce

1 small can organic tomato paste

1 tbsp pineapple juice

(juice naturally from an organic pineapple)

1 tsp minced garlic

1 tbsp onion powder

1 tsp pepper

1 ½ tsp salt

3 packets Stevia

1 ½ tbsp hot sauce (organic, no syrups or starches, made with apple cider vinegar)

Brown grown beef, drain, combine all ingredients, and serve with roasted broccoli

Grass Fed Meatloaf

2 ½ lbs ground grass fed beef

3 cups chopped yellow onion

2 tsp fresh thyme leaves chopped

½ tbsp salt and pepper

2 tbsps Annie's Worcestershire sauce

1 tbsp tomato paste

½ cup gluten-free bread crumbs

2 egg whites

1 cup Organicvalley Agave Ketchup

Mix it all together. Form loaf. Lay on cooling rack sitting inside a half sheet pan. Cover the top with Organicvalley Agave Ketchup. About a cup. Cook at 350°F for 70 minutes

Melt in your Mouth Roast

3 lb Rump Roast. Grass fed organic beef

Sea salt, garlic powder, pepper to taste

1 tbsp olive oil

2 tbsp organic Worcestershire sauce (made with agave found at Whole Foods)

1 large white organic onion

Tall crock pot – not large oval

Cut roast in half; add salt, pepper and garlic powder to each side of the roast. Place olive oil in a skillet and brown each side of the roast lightly. Cut onion in large slices. Place onion at the bottom of the crock pot. After browning the roast, set it side by side in the crock pot. It will be a tight fit, laying it on top of the onions. Take the remaining drippings and deglaze the pan with the 2 tbsps of Worcestershire sauce. Stir for 2 minutes and poor on top of the roast. Cook on high for 20 mins and on low for 5 hours. The roast should fall apart. Strain onions and you can serve it with the roast. YUMMMMM!!!!!

BISON

Agave Chili Sauce Bison Burger

1 ½ lbs bison

Cayenne pepper

1 bottle minced onion

Annie's Organic Worcestershire sauce

Organicville Agave Ketchup

1 tbsp tomato paste

2 Stevia Packets

1 tbsp minced garlic

1 ½ tbsp Bragg's Liquid Aminos

Chili Sauce:

Make chili sauce with ½ bottle agave ketchup, 1 tbsp tomato paste, 1 tsp cayenne pepper, ½ jar minced onion, 1 tbsp agave nectar, ¼ cup worcestershire sauce, 2 Stevia packets. Combine all ingredients together and add salt and pepper to taste.

Pour on top of bison and mix together well. Form patties and cook on the grill until pink color disappears (George Foreman or grill pans work as well). Measure out 3 oz each day for patties. The caramelized onions taste great on top as well!

Bison Beef Stew

2 lbs bison

Sea salt

Pepper

2 tbsps olive oil

4 carrots

1 white onion

1 bunch celery

1 sweet potato

1 can organic green beans

2 cans whole organic tomato

2 cups button mushrooms, halved

1 tsp thyme

1 tsp dried red pepper

1 tbsp brown rice flour

1 tsp parsley

1 full clove garlic minced

28 oz low-sodium organic beef broth

Mix bison, salt, pepper, and flour together well and refrigerate for 10 minutes. Heat a soup pan on high heat until it is preheated. Add the olive oil and then add the meat. Brown on each side for about 1 minute. Then add mushroom, onion, and celery. Cook for about 8 minutes or until onions are cooked down well. Add carrots and remaining veggies except sweet potato along with beef broth. Bring to a boil uncovered on high. Then cover and cook for 45 minutes. Add sweet potato. Cover and cook for 1 hour.

BBQ Bison Meatloaf

2 lbs ground bison

1 full bunch celery, chopped

1 whole red pepper, chopped

1 whole green pepper, chopped

1 whole white onion, chopped

2 tbsps tomato paste

2 jars Bone Suckin' BBQ Sauce

2 carrots, chopped

Olive oil

1 tbsp minced garlic

1 tsp pepper

1 tsp salt

1 tsp cayenne pepper

Sautee all veggies in olive oil. Combine all ingredients, including 1 whole jar Bone Suckin' BBQ Sauce and form a meatloaf. Set on top of cooking rack and set inside a roasting pan for proper drainage. Pour half of the other jar of Bone Suckin' BBQ Sauce over the loaf and cook on 375°F for 50 minutes. Coat with more sauce and cook for 25 minutes at 350. Turn off the oven and leave the meatloaf in there for another 20-30 minutes until done in the center.

Bison Chili

1/4 cup extra-virgin olive oil

2 pounds bison stew meat

1 cup diced white onion

1 cup diced carrots

1 cup diced celery

3 cloves garlic, minced

1/2 cup tomato paste

4 cups organic free-range low-sodium beef broth

1 (14.5-ounce) can chopped tomatoes

Salt and freshly ground black pepper

4 tablespoons chopped parsley leaves

2 teaspoons chopped thyme leaves

Heat the oil in a large saucepan over medium-high heat, until almost smoking. Brown the bison meat in the hot oil until golden brown, then remove from the pan to a plate and set aside. In the same pan, add the onion, carrots, celery, garlic and saute for about 5 minutes, stirring constantly. Add tomato paste and stir well. Slowly add in the beef stock and canned tomatoes. Season with salt and pepper, to taste. Return the seared meat to the pan and reduce the heat to a simmer. Stir in the fresh herbs and continue to cook for about 45 minutes. It will be done when the fluid volume has reduced by approximately half.

Bison Crock Pot Sirloin

Season 3 lbs of bison sirloin with Debbie's Seasoning. Set inside of a tall not wide crock pot. Top with 3 tbsp of Schutlz's Gourmet Hot Sauce. Cook on low for 8 hours. Drain the liquid and shred the meat. Tastes great with more hot sauce on top when you eat. Schutlz's Gourmet Hot Sauce is available at Whole Foods. Bison Sirloin is available at Whole Foods, as well. YUM!

Bison Flank Steak

4 lbs bison flank steak
2 tbsps extra-virgin olive oil
Sea salt and pepper

Preheat the oven to 400°F. Rub the olive oil, salt, and pepper all over bison. Place on a cookie sheet lined with foil. Roast about 20-25 minutes, flipping once.

BBQ Bison Roast

5 lbs Bison Chuck Roast

Season liberally with pepper, garlic powder, onion powder and a dash of cayenne. Top with 2 tbsp Schutlz's Gourmet Hot Sauce. Place in crock pot. Cook on high 1 hour and low 8-10 hours. Shred meat and add 1 bottle Bone Suckin' BBQ Sauce.

Bison Roast

5 lbs bison chuck roast, trimmed
Garlic powder
Onion powder
2 tbsps Shultz's Gourmet Hot Sauce

Set a crockpot to high and place the roast in the crockpot. Rub the entire roast generously with garlic and onion powder, then pour 2 tbsp Shultz's Gourmet Hot Sauce on top (can be found at Whole Foods). Cook on high for 1 hour then reduce to low and cook for an additional 5-7 hours, depending on desired doneness. Shred the roast with a fork and mix in 1/4 cup low-sodium vegetable broth and 1 tbsp olive oil to keep it moist.

Grilled Bison Sirloin Steak

Mix pepper, garlic powder, onion powder and a small amount of cayenne together based on the size of your meat. Equal parts of each except cayenne. Brush your steak with olive oil and rub with seasoning. Warm your skillet on medium. Cook until desired doneness and per the size of the steak. Medium would be a temperature of about 120°F or 7-10 minutes on each side. Let the steak rest under foil for at least 5 minutes after.

French Onion Bison Beef Tips

2 lbs bison (chopped like stew meat)

1 tbsp organic olive oil

1 tbsp organic minced garlic

2 whole organic white onions

1 quart organic low-sodium vegetable broth

½ jar Annie's Organic Worcestershire Sauce

Brown the bison in a skillet with 1 tablespoon olive oil. Slice the onions and place them on the bottom of a crockpot with 1 tablespoon garlic. Place the meat on top and pour in the low-sodium vegetable broth and Worcestershire sauce. Roast on low approximately 6 to 10 hours (overnight). Roast longer for increased tenderness and flavor.

*Beef stock or French onion soup may be substituted for the vegetable broth.
*Grass-fed beef will produce a more tender cut due to the fat and may be substituted for bison.

Hulkburger

4 lbs ground bison

1 bottle Organicville Agave Ketchup

1 bottle minced onion

Sauce:

½ bottle Organicville Agave Ketchup

1 bottle minced onion

1 tbsp garlic powder

1 tsp cayenne

1 tbsp dry mustard

2 packets Stevia

1 tbsp apple cider vinegar

Preheat the oven to 400°F. On a flat surface, spread the bison flat and mix in ketchup and minced onion. Form even 6oz patties and place on a drying rack. Mix all of the ingredients together for the sauce in a large bowl and spoon on top of each burger. Line the bottom of the oven rack with foil and place the burgers on the cooling rack in the oven. Bake on 400°F for 40 minutes. If you like them more done like a meatloaf, turn off oven and let them sit for another 20-30 minutes. Remove the burgers from the oven and let cool. Place each in a container for meals throughout the day. Cooking them this way allows the fat to drain easily and makes clean up a breeze!

Roasted Bison Flank Steak

5 lbs bison flank steak

Season it with garlic powder, onion powder, pepper and cayenne. Fold them in half and lay them on their sides next to each other. Cook them in crockpot on high for an hour and low for 6 hours. Shreds apart.

Shredded BBQ Bison Roast

4 lbs bison chuck roast

1 tsp garlic powder

1 tsp onion powder

1 tsp celery salt

1 tbsp Schultz's Gourmet Hot Sauce

1 tbsp Liquid Smoke (optional)

1 jar Bone Suckin' BBQ Sauce

Set a slow cooker on low heat for 6-8 hours. Place bison chuck roast in the slow cooker and rub the garlic powder, onion powder, and celery salt on the roast. Drizzle on the hot sauce and Liquid Smoke and cover. Cook for 6-8 hours or until the meat is tender and shreds apart with a fork. Strain the juices and shred the roast. Place it in a nonstick skillet, add the BBQ sauce and warm on low for 5 minutes. Separate into portions for the week. This recipe is so yummy you could die! Way better than any pulled pork sandwich.

Spicy Bison Stew

2 lbs cubed bison stew meat

2 green peppers

1 orange or yellow pepper

1 large onion

2 tbsps minced garlic

1 bay leaf

3 cups chopped tomatoes. Fresh if not canned will do

2 tbsps cumin

2 tbsps chili powder

½ tbsp cayenne pepper

1 tbsp red pepper flakes

Sauce meat in a large dutch oven in olive oil. Remove meat and sauce the onion and garlic, then add peppers and tomatoes and spices let cook down then add meat back in. Salt and pepper to taste. Cook for 2.5 hours on low with lid on. Add 1/2 cup regular coffee and cook on low for another hour. Whole Foods will cut the bison roast meat for you. Call ahead. Recipe courtesy of Ina Garten.

FISH

Agave Grilled Salmon

Four 5 oz pieces of Salmon

Agave Nectar

Brush about a tsp of agave nectar on each side of the salmon. Warm a grill pan with 1 tbsp olive oil; on medium heat place all four pieces of salmon on grill pan and there should be a sizzle. Cook on each side for 5 to 7 minutes. Agave will caramelize and be so delicious you might die.

Baked Balsamic Pineapple Salmon

1 ½ lbs salmon

3 tbsp olive oil

2 tsp apple cider vinegar

2 tsp balsamic vinegar

2 tbsp pineapple juice

2 packets Stevia

1 tsp minced garlic

1 tbsp canola oil

Spread canola oil in a baking dish. spread salt, pepper, and garlic across the top of the salmon. Mix olive oil, vinegars, pineapple juice and Stevia and whisk together well. Pour the liquid over the salmon. Bake at 350°F for 17 minutes. Turn on the broiler and cook for 3 minutes to caramelize the flavor on top and add a little crunch.

Baked Cod

Baste cod with olive oil, garlic powder, onion powder, pepper and a dash of cayenne pepper. Set a cooling rack inside a baking dish. Set cod on top of baking dish. Cook at 350°F for 25 minutes.

Cranberry Pineapple Salmon

Four 5 oz pieces of Salmon

3 tbsp agave nectar

1 tbsp olive oil

1 bag frozen cranberries

1 can no-sugar added crushed pineapple

Brush about a tsp of agave nectar on each side of the salmon. Warm a grill pan with 1 tbsp olive oil; on medium heat place all four pieces of salmon on grill pan and there should be a sizzle. Cook on each side for 5 to 7 minutes. Agave will caramelize and be so delicious you might die. Warm the cranberries on medium heat in a nonstick skillet. Drain and rinse the pineapple and add to cranberries in the sauce pan after it has cooled. Place 1 ½ tbsp cranberry pineapple mixture on top of each piece of salmon.

Crunchy Lemon-Pepper Grilled Salmon

2 lbs organic salmon, skinned

Salt-free lemon pepper seasoning (Mrs. Dash for example)

2 tbsp olive oil

Cover salmon in lemon-pepper seasoning and olive oil. Spray a grill pan with olive oil spray and warm on medium heat for 4 minutes so the salmon sears when it is placed on the pan. Cook on one side for 5 minutes, baste the other side with more olive oil and flip. Cook for an additional 5 minutes until desired doneness. It is really good crispy and crunchy

Mustard Encrusted Tilapia

3 tbsp Annie's Dijon Mustard (organic found at Whole foods – no corn syrup or starches and made with apple cider vinegar)

1 tbsp Annie's German Mustard (same as above)

2 tbsps minced shallots (can use garlic)

1 tbsp organic olive oil

1 tbsp apple cider vinegar (I use BRAGGS brand)

Salt and Pepper both sides of the tilapia. Spray a nonstick skillet with organic olive oil spray. Lightly brown each side of the filets. Spray a baking dish, spread mixture onto the filet, bake in dish for 10 mins on 325°F, set under broiler for 2 mins.

Lemon Garlic Tilapia

Foil line a roasting pan. Season 6 tilapia fillet's with sea salt, pepper, garlic powder and onion powder evenly. Add a dash of cayenne on top. Thin slice lemons and lay 2 slices on top of each tilapia filet. Cook uncovered at 350°F for 20 minutes. Then cover with foil and cook for 15 more.

Pan-Seared Ezekiel Bread Crumb Encrusted Tilapia

5 pieces of Ezekiel bread

3 lbs tilapia filets

Olive Oil

Salt and pepper

1 ½ tsp paprika

1 tbsp parsley

1 ½ tbsp dried minced onion

3 egg whites

Set 5 pieces of Ezekiel bread out over night. The next day crumble the bread onto a cookie sheet. I used a food processor to crumble it. Add 1 tsp salt and 1 tsp pepper, paprika, parsley and minced onion to the breadcrumb mixture and mix together. Bake the bread crumbs at 300°F for 10 mins. Set aside to cool. Salt and pepper the tilapia, then run it through the egg whites and cover it with the bread crumbs. Warm the skillet over medium heat with 2 to 3 tbsp olive oil in it. Drop the tilapia in the olive oil, there should be a sizzle. Cook for 4 to 8 minutes on each side. I just keep flipping it every 2 minutes for about 12 minutes. Let cool on a wire rack and pat out any extra oil with a paper

Pan-Seared Tilapia

3 lbs tilapia filets

3 tbsps extra-virgin olive oil

2 tbsps garlic powder

2 tbsps onion powder

1 tsp sea salt

1 tsp pepper

1 tsp cayenne peppers

Heat a grill pan on medium-high heat and coat with olive oil. Place tilapia filets on the grill pan and season one side. Cook about 5 minutes on one side, flip and coat the other side with seasoning. Cook an additional 5 minutes. Flip once more and cook an additional 2-5 minutes per side until desired crispiness.

Pan-Seared Tuna Steak Salad

Tuna Steak:

1 ½ lbs tuna steak

1 tsp minced garlic

Salt and pepper

Organic olive oil cooking spray

Rub the minced garlic, salt and pepper onto each side of the tuna steak. Spray a nonstick cooking skillet with the cooking spray. Cook each side of the tuna steak for 5 minutes. Take tuna off the heat and place a lid on top of the skillet. Let it sit in the skillet off the heat and cook further for at least 5 minutes.

Mustard Vinaigrette:

3 tbsp apple cider vinegar

½ tsp dijon mustard

½ tsp minced garlic

1 tbsp olive-oil mayonnaise

1 tsp salt

¼ tsp pepper

$1/3$ cup olive oil

2 packets Stevia

Whisk ingredients together in large bowl. Chop up and combine with mustard vinaigrette, celery, and red grapes. Chop up tuna and combine with red grapes, celery, and mixed greens. Drizzle vinaigrette on top.

Roasted Salmon and Asparagus Salad

Roasted Salmon:

Salt and pepper Salmon. Spray a baking dish with olive oil spray. Combine 1 tbsp pineapple juice from organic canned pineapple, 1 tbsp organic balsamic vinegar, 1 tbsp apple cider vinegar, 1 tbsp olive oil and 2 Stevia packets and pour over the top of the salmon. Bake at 325°F for 12 mins, 3 mins under the broiler.

Roasted Asparagus:

Preheat oven to 400°F. Lay asparagus evenly on a sheet with salt and pepper, 1 tsp garlic powder, 1 tsp onion powder, and 1 ½ tbsp organic olive oil. Bake for 15 – 20 mins until it's tender yet crisp.

Salmon Salad

2 lbs cooked salmon, chilled

1 cup small-diced celery (3 stalks)

½ cup small-diced red onion (1 small onion)

2 tbsps minced fresh dill

2 tbsps raspberry vinegar

2 tbsps organic extra-virgin olive oil

½ tsp kosher salt

½ tsp freshly ground black pepper

Break the salmon into very large flakes, removing any skin and bones, and place the salmon in a bowl. Add the celery, red onion, dill, raspberry vinegar, olive oil, salt, and pepper. Season to taste. Mix well and serve cold or at room temperature.

Seasoned Tilapia

Brush tilapia sparingly with olive oil. Combine equal amounts of pepper, garlic powder, and onion powder with a small amount of cayenne and rub onto tilapia.

Brush olive oil across a foil lined baking sheet so fish does not stick. Bake fish at 350°F for 20 minutes flipping 1 time in between, or until desired doneness

Tilapia Salad

Tilapia:

1 ½ lbs tilapia

1 ½ tbsps olive oil

Mustard Dressing:

1 ½ tbsps olive oil

Salt & Pepper

2 tbsps ground organic mustard

2 tbsps organic Dijon mustard

2 tbsps apple cider vinegar

2 packets Stevia

2 cups celery, chopped

¾ white onion

Salt and pepper tilapia. Heat a nonstick skillet on medium with olive oil. Add fish when oil is so hot it causes fish to sizzle. Brown on each side until crunchy. Flake apart all of the filets in a big bowl. Whisk dressing ingredients together thoroughly. Combine celery, onion and tilapia in a large bowl and drizzle dressing over the top. Mix well.

POULTRY

Chicken Chili

1 pound ground chicken breast

1 whole green pepper

1 whole red pepper

2 garlic cloves

1 stalk celery

5 large carrots

1 small can tomato paste

1 large can chunk tomatoes

Mrs. Dash Extra Spicy Seasoning Blend

Cook chicken in pan with seasoning to taste on medium-high heat coated with olive oil cooking spray. Once cooked, add peppers and cook on medium. Then add the garlic, celery, and carrots. When these ingredients are cooked, add tomatoes and tomato paste. Let simmer on low for at least 30 minutes.

Debbie's Seasoned Chicken

Lay 6 boneless, skinless chicken breasts in a baking pan. Brush with olive oil on both sides and season with Debbie's seasoning on both sides. Sprinkle oregano over the top of the chicken breasts. Cook at 350°F for 40 minutes. Cover with foil and rest for 10 minutes.

Debbie's Seasoning:

Into an empty shaker add 2 tsps cayenne, 2 tbps granulated garlic, 2 tbsps granulated onion, 1 tbsp black pepper, 1 tbsps sea salt. Shake on anything. Tastes great.

Chicken Fingers

½ cup sliced almonds

¼ cup oat flour

1 ½ tsps paprika

½ tsp garlic powder

½ tsp onion powder

½ tsp dry mustard

Salt and pepper

4 large egg whites

1 pound chicken tenders

Olive oil cooking spray

Preheat oven to 475°F. Line a baking sheet with foil. Set a wire rack on the baking sheet and coat it with cooking spray. Place almonds, oat flour, paprika, garlic powder, onion powder, dry mustard, salt and pepper in a food processor; process until the almonds are finely chopped and the paprika is mixed throughout, about 1 minute. Transfer the mixture to a shallow dish. Whisk egg whites in a second shallow dish. Add chicken tenders and turn to coat. Transfer each tender to the almond mixture; turn to coat evenly. (Discard any remaining egg white and almond mixture.) Place the tenders on the prepared rack and coat with cooking spray; turn and spray the other side. Bake the chicken fingers until golden brown, crispy and no longer pink in the center, 20 to 25 minutes.

Crunchy Chicken Dijon

4 grilled chicken cutlets, pounded flat

2 tbsps Annie's Dijon Mustard

2 tbsps olive oil

2 tbsps water

6 pieces Ezekiel bread, toasted

1 tbsp garlic powder

1 tbsp onion powder

1 tbsp parsley

½ tsp cayenne pepper

2 tsps black pepper

Put the pieces of bread in a food processor with garlic powder, onion powder, parsley, cayenne, and black pepper. Blend until the bread is an even crumb mixture, spread evenly over a baking sheet, and cook for 10 minutes at 400°F.

Combine the mustard, water, olive oil, and additional pepper (if desired) in a flat pan. Dredge chicken breasts through this mixture then through the bread crumbs. Lay a cooling rack on top of a roasting pan and place the chicken on the cooling rack. Cook at 400°F for about 25 minutes.

Ezekiel Bread Crumb Encrusted Chicken Cutlet

5 pieces Ezekiel bread

4 boneless, skinless chicken breasts butterflied
   and pounded flat

Olive Oil

Salt and pepper

1 ½ tsp cayenne pepper

1 tbsp parsley

1 ½ tbsps dried minced onion

3 egg whites

Set 5 pieces of Ezekiel bread out over night. The next day, crumble the bread onto a cookie sheet. I used a food processor to crumble it. Add 1 tsp salt and 1 tsp pepper, cayenne pepper, parsley and minced onion to the breadcrumb mixture and mix together. Bake the bread crumbs at 300°F for 10 mins. Set aside to cool. Pound out chicken until flat. It is easier if you have it butter flied first or just buy it that way. Then, still pound it out more even if it is butter flied. Salt and pepper the chicken, run it through the egg whites and then run it through the bread crumbs. Warm the skillet over medium heat with 2 to 3 tbsp olive oil in it. Drop the chicken in the olive oil, there should be a sizzle. Cook for 4 to 8 minutes on each side. I just keep flipping it every 2 minutes for about 12 minutes. Let cool on a wire rack and pat out any extra oil with a paper towel.

This is so much better than having rice as your carb or bread for a sandwich. It is well worth the time it takes. I take the agave ketchup that I use and add hot sauce to it to make a dipping sauce for the chicken. It is delicious. Whole Foods has the agave ketchup whish is free of all syrups and fillers. They also have hot sauce which is free of the same.

Grilled Chicken Wing Cutlets

3 large boneless, skinless chicken breasts

1 tbsp garlic powder

1 tbsp onion powder

2 cups low-sodium vegetable stock

2 cups water

1 jar Shultz Gourmet Hot Sauce

Set a slow cooker on low heat for 6-8 hours. Line the bottom of the cooker with the breasts and sprinkle with garlic and onion powder. Add the low-sodium chicken broth and water to completely cover the chicken breasts. Cook on low for 6-8 hours, until the chicken is tender and shreds apart with a fork. Drain the liquid and shred the chicken. Place the shredded chicken back in the slow cooker, add the hot sauce and mix well. Let the chicken sit on warm for a few minutes before dividing into portions for the week.

Lemon Chicken

½ cup olive oil

Add 3 tbsp garlic and the oil in a sauce pan, add 1 lemon zested, 2 tbsp fresh lemon juice, 1 1/2 taps dried oregano, 1tsp fresh thyme, 1tbsp salt. Pour it into a baking dish, lay 4 chicken breasts seasoned with salt and pepper. Brush them with olive oil. Cut an entire lemon into wedges and roast in the dish with the chicken. Cook at 400°F for 40 minutes. Wrap with foil when you remove. Let rest for 10 minutes. Serve on rice

Hot Chicken Salad

2 cups cooked chicken breast, cubed

1 ½ cups diced celery

½ cup slivered almonds

½ tsp onion powder

½ tsp garlic powder

¼ tsp black pepper

¼ tsp cayenne pepper

2 tbsps fresh –squeezed lemon juice

1 cup omega (olive-oil based) mayonnaise

1 cup toasted Ezekiel bread crumbs

Spray a 13x9 inch pan with olive oil cooking spray and preheat the oven to 375°F. Combine all of the ingredients except the breadcrumbs in a bowl and spread it evenly on the bottom of the pan. Layer the bread crumbs on top of the chicken mixture and bake for 30-40 minutes. Remove from the oven and let cool before dividing into portions for the week. Recipe inspired by Paula Dean.

Lemon Garlic Roasted Turkey Breast

5 - 7 lb turkey breast with skin

2 tbsps olive oil

1 tbsp minced garlic

2 tbsps lemon juice

2 tsps dry mustard

1 tsp rosemary

1 tsp sage

1 tsp onion powder

½ tsp pepper

¾ cup low sodium vegetable stock

Preheat oven to 325°F. Place turkey breast on a rack in a roasting pan skin side up.

Combine all ingredients except vegetable stock and under the skin of the turkey. Pot stock into the bottom of the pan. Brush 1 teaspoon olive oil over skin. Check the breast after an hour and if its over-browned, cover it loosely with foil. Cook for another 30 to 40 minutes. Allow it to set at room temperature for at least 15 minutes.

Remove skin and toss. Slice the turkey up ahead of time.

Roasted BBQ Chicken

3 large boneless, skinless chicken breasts

1 tbsp garlic powder

1 tbsp onion powder

2 cups low-sodium vegetable stock

2 cups water

1 jar Bone Suckin' BBQ Sauce

Set a slow cooker on low heat for 6-8 hours. Line the bottom of the cooker with the breasts and sprinkle with garlic and onion powder. Add the low-sodium chicken broth and water to completely cover the chicken breasts. Cook on low for 6-8 hours, until the chicken is tender and shreds apart with a fork. Drain the liquid and shred the chicken. Place the shredded chicken back in the slow cooker, add the BBQ sauce and mix well. Let the chicken sit on warm for a few minutes before dividing into portions for the week.

Shredded BBQ Chicken

7 boneless, skinless chicken breasts

Water or chicken stock

1 jar Bone Suckin' BBQ Sauce

Put breasts in crock pot and fill crockpot with water or chicken broth to the top. Cook on low for 6 hours. Drain all liquid and shred chicken with fork. Add 1 bottle of Bone Suckin' Sauce to the shredded chicken and mix!

BBQ Chicken

3 bone in skin on chicken breasts

Olive oil

Salt and pepper

Lay chicken skin side up in a shallow baking dish, sprinkle salt and pepper and drizzle with olive oil. Cook for 45 to 50 minutes in a 350°F oven. Remove from bone and skin, and then mix with barbecue sauce.

Barbecue Sauce:

1 ½ cups chopped yellow onion (1 large onion)

1 tbsp minced garlic (3 cloves)

$^1/_3$ cup organic extra-virgin olive oil

1 cup tomato paste (10 oz)

1 cup apple cider vinegar

¼ cup agave nectar

½ cup worcestershire sauce

1 cup dijon mustard

½ cup low sodium soy sauce

2 tbsps chili powder

1 tbsp ground cumin

½ tbsp crushed red pepper flakes

In a large saucepan on low heat, sauté the onions and garlic with the olive oil for 10 to 15 minutes, until the onions are translucent, but not browned. Add the tomato paste, vinegar, agave, worcestershire sauce, mustard, soy sauce, chili powder, cumin, and red pepper flakes. Simmer uncovered on low heat for 30 minutes. Use immediately or store in the refrigerator.

Spicy Chicken Wingettes

4 lbs chicken breast tenderloins

1 cup Schultz's Gourmet Hot Sauce
   (or other clean hot sauce)

¼ cup locally harvested honey

1 tbsp olive oil, extra for chicken

1 tbsp garlic powder + extra for chicken

1 tbsp onion powder + extra for chicken

1 tsp paprika

Preheat oven to 350°F. Place chicken breast tenderloins on a roasting pan lined with foil and sprinkle with garlic and onion powder. Drizzle olive oil over chicken tenderloins and ensure they are evenly coated. Cover the chicken with another piece of foil so that they are not exposed to the oven. Bake the chicken for 50 minutes. Combine all the other ingredients for the sauce in a bowl. Remove the top layer of foil and pour out any excess liquid. Pour the sauce evenly over the chicken tenderloins. Ensure they are evenly coated on both sides, turn the oven to broil and cook an additional 10 minutes.

Spicy Orange Chicken

Heat up ⅓ cup olive oil and add 1 teaspoon cayenne, 1 teaspoon sea salt. ½ cup orange juice from the orange and the zest of a full orange. Spread across a 9x9 pan. Lay 6 chicken breasts on top. Brush the top of the chicken breasts with olive oil and sprinkle sea salt and pepper to taste on top. Cook at 350°F for 45 minutes. Remove from oven, cover with foil and let rest for 10 minutes.

Grain-Free Turkey Meatloaf

3 lbs ground turkey

1 bottle Organicville Agave Ketchup

1 tsp pepper

1 tsp garlic powder

1 tsp onion powder

1 tsp minced onion

1 tsp cayenne pepper

1 chopped onion

1 full bunch of chopped celery

Mix half of the bottle of ketchup with the rest of the ingredients. Set a cooling rack inside a shallow foil-lined roasting pan. Form the loaf on top of the cooling rack and top with the other half of ketchup. Cook at 350°F for 90 minutes.

Turkey Meatloaf

2 lbs lean ground turkey

1 ½ large yellow onion, chopped

1 cup thin chopped celery

2 tbsps organic tomato paste

½ cup Annie's Organic Worcestershire Sauce

⅓ cup organic free-range chicken stock

1 whole organic egg

1 cup organic whole oats

1 cup Organicville Agave Ketchup

Sauté onion and celery, and then cool. Combine all ingredients except ketchup and form a loaf onto a baking sheet with sides. Lining the sheets with foil makes cleaning easier.. Add ketchup to the top.

Cook for 1 hour 30 minutes at 325°F. Turn oven off and let remain in oven for 10 more minutes.

Whole Oven-Baked Chicken

5 lb roasting chicken

Sea salt

Black pepper

2 lemons

4 cloves of garlic

2 ½ tbsps olive oil

1 large onion thinly sliced

1 cup chicken stock

Preheat oven 425°F. Remove giblets. Pat dry the chicken. Place cut up garlic and lemon inside the chicken. Brush the chicken with olive oil and sprinkle with sea salt and pepper. Tie the legs together and tuck the wings. Place in small roasting pan. Place onions in bowl and toss them with 1/2 tablespoon olive oil, sea salt and pepper. Surround the chicken with onions. Pour the chicken stock onto the bottom of the roasting pan. Cook for an hour and 20 minutes then remove from oven and immediately cover with foil. Let rest for 10 minutes. Remove all skin and all meat from the bone. Throw out the skin and store all the meat together.

VEGGIES

Baked Green Beans

5 steam in bag green beans

4 tbsp extra virgin olive oil

1 tbsp pepper

Cook all bags together in microwave for 25 minutes. Spread across foil lined sheetcake pan. Hand kneed the olive oil so that all beans are covered. Sprinkle pepper over the top. Cook for 40 minutes on 350. Turn oven off and let rest in oven for 5 to 10 more minutes or until desired.

Baked Sweet Potatoes

Foil line a baking sheet. Lay 7 sweet potatoes out on the sheet. Cook for 90 minutes on 400°F. Let cool and store covered in fridge with skin intact. Pull skin off 1 sweet potato daily and measure out desired amount.

Caramelized Balsamic Onions

2 white onions

Balsamic vinegar

Olive oil

Warm a large sauté pan with 1 ½ tablespoon olive oil. Slice onions and place into skillet. Make sure onions are all evenly covered with balsamic vinegar. Cook on medium to medium-low heat for 30 minutes minimum. The longer they cook the better they taste.

Chow Chow

4 peeled tomatoes

2 de-seeded cucumbers

1 sliced red onion

1 sliced banana pepper

1 tbsp BRAGG's apple cider vinegar

2 packets Stevia

Salt and pepper

Combine all ingredients together in a bowl and toss with apple cider vinegar and Stevia. Sprinkle salt and pepper to taste on top.

Crisp Citrus Salad

1 large serving Organic Girl spring mix (approx. 3 cups)

1 organic apple, sliced

1 tbsp slivered almonds

1 tsp extra-virgin olive oil

1 packet Stevia

Grapefruit Salad

1 large serving Organic Girl spring mix (approx. 3 cups)

1 organic grapefruit, sliced

1 tbsp slivered almonds

1 tsp extra-virgin olive oil

1 tsp organic lemon juice

1 tbsp apple cider vinegar

Cole Slaw

2 sacks organic slaw mix

⅓ cup olive oil omega-3 mayo

1 tbsp BRAGG's apple cider vinegar

1 tbsp lemon juice

1 tbsp onion powder

1 tbsp pepper

½ tsp cayenne pepper

1 tbsp Annie's Dijon Mustard

1 cup finely diced celery

1 cup finely diced carrots

½ cup finely diced white onion

Combine mayo and the next 8 ingredients in a bowl. Combine lettuce, carrots, celery and onion in a bowl and toss with dressing.

Kale Chips

2 containers pre-chopped kale

2 tbsp extra-virgin olive oil

Salt and pepper

Preheat the oven to 350°F. Spread the kale in an even layer on a cookie sheet lined with aluminum foil. Drizzle the olive oil over the kale and add salt and pepper to taste. Bake for 20 minutes or until the kale becomes crispy. Remove and let cool. These are way better than potato chips and are so yummy!

Lemon Pepper Roasted Broccoli

2 lbs organic broccoli florets

1 zest of whole lemon

Juice of whole lemon

1 tbsp pepper

2 tbsp extra-virgin olive oil

Mix all ingredients in a bowl and knead with hands so all pieces are coated evenly. Place the broccoli in a roasting pan and bake at 400°F for 20 minutes.

Mashed Cauliflower

3 bags frozen cauliflower

2 tbsps Annie's Organic Balsamic Vinegar and Olive Oil dressing

Steam cauliflower in microwave and add to food processor with the dressing. Mash in food processor.

Mashed Sweet Potato

6 medium sweet potatoes

Cinnamon and Stevia

1 tbsp agave nectar

1 tbsp unsweetened almond milk

Preheat oven to 400°F. Wash sweet potatoes and lay on a cookie sheet. Bake for 90 minutes. Remove from oven and let cool. Peel off the skin and mash the sweet potatoes in a bowl. Add agave nectar, almond milk, and more cinnamon and Stevia to taste. Blend with a hand mixer until smooth.

Roasted Asparagus

5 lbs of Fresh Organic Asparagus

Sea Salt and Pepper to taste

4 tbsp Organic Olive Oil

Wash asparagus. Pour out on a large sheet cake pan evenly in one layer. Pour olive oil over the asparagus, salt and pepper to taste. Take your hands and blend it all together and spread it evenly in one layer. Roast on 425°F for 20 to 25 mins or until tips start turning brown. .

Roasted Balsamic Asparagus

5 lbs of Fresh Organic Asparagus

Sea Salt and Pepper to taste

4tbsp Organic Olive Oil

¼ cup Balsamic Vinegar

Wash asparagus. Pour out on a large sheet cake pan evenly in one layer. Pour olive oil over the asparagus, salt and pepper to taste. Take your hands and blend it all together and spread it evenly in one layer. Drizzle balsamic vinegar evenly over asparagus. Roast on 425°F for 20 to 25 mins or until tips start turning brown.

Roasted Carrots

30 organic whole carrots

3 tbsp olive oil

Sea Salt and Pepper

Peel carrots. Slice diagonally into smaller, even pieces. Spread evenly on pan and sprinkle with Stevia, salt, pepper and olive oil. Roast in a 425°F oven for 40-50 minutes.

Roasted Broccoli

4 lbs organic broccoli florets

4 tbsps extra-virgin olive oil

4 cloves garlic, thinly sliced

1 ½ tsps salt

½ tsp pepper

2 tsps grated organic lemon zest

2 tbsps fresh organic lemon juice

1 tsp onion powder

Preheat the oven to 425°F. Line a sheet cake pain with foil. Spread broccoli in a single layer over the pan and add drizzle with olive oil. Sprinkle garlic, salt, pepper, and onion powder evenly over broccoli. Roast for 20 to 25 minutes until crisp and some tips are browned. Immediately add zest, juice and 1 ½ tablespoon olive oil and toss. Oh this makes broccoli taste like candy!!!!!

Roasted Broccoli with Garlic

5 lbs organic broccoli florets

1 ½ tbsp organic minced garlic

Sea salt and pepper

4 tbsps extra-virgin olive oil

Pour broccoli florets out on a large sheet cake pan evenly in one layer. Pour olive oil over the broccoli. Sprinkle garlic, salt, and pepper to taste over broccoli. Roast on 425°F for 20 to 25 minutes or until tips start turning brown.

Roasted Red Peppers

Core and slice 3 red peppers. Toss them in olive oil, salt and pepper. Cook on a foil-lined baking sheet on 350°F for 20 minutes or until desired doneness.

Roasted Red Pepper and Red Onion

Thick slice the peppers and onions, rub them with olive oil, garlic, salt and pepper and roast on a shallow roasting dish at 400°F for 20 minutes.

Roasted Tomatoes

25 plum tomatoes (aka Roma) halved and
   seeds removed

5 tbsp extra-virgin olive oil

2 cloves garlic, minced

Salt and pepper

3 Stevia packets

1/3 cup balsamic vinegar

Spread the tomato halves evenly across a sheet cake pan. Drizzle each with olive oil, salt, pepper, Stevia, and balsamic vinegar. Roast at 450°F for 25 to 30 minutes until caramelized.

Roasted Zucchini

6-8 zucchini

Salt and Pepper

3-4 tbsps extra-virgin olive oil

Thick slice zucchini and spread evenly across a sheet cake pan. Drizzle with olive oil, salt, and pepper. Roast at 400°F for 20 minutes.

Spaghetti Squash

1 large spaghetti squash

Extra-virgin olive oil

Microwave the squash for 2 minutes. Remove and cut in half with a large, sturdy kitchen knife. Scoop out seeds with a large spoon. Preheat oven to 400°F. Drizzle olive oil over squash and lay face down on a cookie sheet. Roast for 40 minutes, remove and shred with a fork while still warm.

BREAKFAST

Apple Cinnamon Pancake

6 egg whites

¾ cup unsweetened organic applesauce

½ tsp cinnamon

1 packet Stevia

1 drop alcohol-free vanilla

Blend all ingredients in a blender. Spray skillet with olive oil. Cook on low to medium heat until set and flip. Cook for another minute. Spread almond butter on top while warm.

Blueberry Banana Pancake

⅓ cup oats

3 egg whites

½ scoop vanilla protein

¼ cup blueberries

½ banana

2 packets Stevia

Blend all ingredients in a blender. Heat a nonstick skillet to medium heat and spray olive oil cooking spray on it. Pour the batter into the skillet and cook until the top is hard, flip and cook an additional minute. So yummy topped with almond butter!

Cinnamon Vanilla Egg White Pancake

6 organic egg whites

1 tbsp organic cinnamon

2 packets Stevia

1 tsp organic alcohol-free vanilla

Combine all ingredients in a blender and blend on medium for 30-45 seconds. Mixture should be frothy like batter. Heat a skillet and spray olive oil non-stick cooking spray on top. Pour egg white mixture into pan and cook on medium for 1 minute or until top is hard. Flip and cook an additional minute.

Egg White French Toast

4 egg whites

2 pieces Ezekiel bread

1/2 tbsp cinnamon

2 packets stevia

Mix egg whites with Stevia, cinnamon, and vanilla in a bowl. Soak the bread in the bowl then fry it in a pan with olive oil. Cook about 2 minutes each side.

Pumpkin Pancake

6 organic egg whites

2 tbsp organic canned pumpkin

1 tbsp cinnamon

2 packets Stevia

1 tsp organic alcohol-free vanilla

Combine all ingredients in a blender and blend until smooth. Heat a nonstick skillet on medium-low heat and spray with olive oil or coconut oil cooking spray. Pour the batter into the skillet and cook until the top begins to bubble. Flip and cook an additional minute. Delicious topped with almond butter and extra cinnamon and Stevia!

Sweet Potato Pancake

1 small sweet potato

6 egg whites

1 tbsp cinnamon

2 packets stevia

Bake the sweet potato on a foil-lined cookie sheet for 90 minutes at 400°F. Remove the skin and mash the sweet potato in a large bowl. Combine with egg whites, cinnamon, and Stevia in a blender and blend until smooth. Spray a skillet with olive oil and cook on medium-low heat until done on one side. Cook on other side for 1 minute and let cool.

Zucchini Pancake

2 medium zucchini (about 3/4 pound)

2 tbsps grated red onion

2 egg whites, beaten

6-8 tbsps brown rice flour

1 tsp baking powder

1 tsp kosher salt

½ tsp freshly ground black pepper

1 tbsp extra-virgin olive oil

Preheat the oven to 300°F.

Grate the zucchini into a bowl using the large grating side of a boxgrater. Immediately stir in the onion and eggs. Stir in 6 tablespoons of the flour, the baking powder, salt, and pepper. (If the batter gets too thin from the liquid in the zucchini, add the remaining 2 tablespoons of flour.)

Heat a large (10 to 12-inch) sauté pan over medium heat and add olive oil. Lower the heat to medium-low and drop heaping soup spoons of batter into the pan. Cook the pancakes about 2 minutes on each side, until browned. Place the pancakes on a sheet pan and keep warm in the oven. Continue to fry the pancakes until all the batter is used. The pancakes can stay warm in the oven for up to 30 minutes. Serve hot.

Strawberry Protein Bar

2 cups quick cook oats

½ cup natural almond butter

4 scoops strawberry Jay Robb egg white protein powder

1 tbsp ground flaxseed

½ cup water

1 tbsp agave

3 packets Stevia

1 cup unsweetened dried strawberries

Knead all ingredients in a large bowl. Line square baking pan with wax paper. Spread dough into pan using a spatula. Optional: Spread a thin layer of peanut butter on top of dough. Freeze for 30 minutes. Remove from freezer & cut into bars.

Vanilla Apricot Protein Bar

2 cups quick cook oats

½ cup natural almond butter

4 scoops vanilla Jay Robb egg white protein powder

1 tbsp ground flaxseed

½ cup water

1 tbsp agave

2 packets Stevia

1 cup unsweetened dried apricots

1 tsp alcohol-free vanilla

Knead all ingredients in a large bowl. Line square baking pan with wax paper. Spread dough into pan using a spatula. Optional: Spread a thin layer of peanut butter on top of dough. Freeze for 30 minutes. Remove from freezer & cut into bars.

Pumpkin Protein Bar

2 cups quick cook oats

½ cup natural peanut butter

4 scoops protein powder (vanilla or cookies & cream)

1 Tbsp ground flaxseed

½ cup water

¾ cup pumpkin

1 tbsp agave

3 packets Stevia

Knead all ingredients in a large bowl. Line square baking pan with wax paper. Spread dough into pan using a spatula. Optional: Spread a thin layer of peanut butter on top of dough. Freeze for 30 minutes. Remove from freezer & cut into bars.

REFERENCES AND SUGGESTED READING

Everyday a Friday - Joel Osteen
Your best Life Now – Joel Osteen
Its your time – Joel Osteen
Become a better you – Joel Osteen
The Four Agreements – Don Miguel Ruiz
Eat Right for your Blood Type – Peter Adamo
Holy Bible – NIV Version

Maxwell Daily Reader – John Maxwell
Make Today Count – John Maxwell
Winning with People – John Maxwell
Today Matters – John Maxwell
Think on These Things – John Maxwell
Dr. Mercola – Website and weekly articles

References

1. Norris J, Messina G. Is It Safe to Eat Soy? Vegan Health. *http://www.veganhealth.org/articles/soymessina.* Accessed July 2010. Skae, T. The Truth About Unfermented Soy and Its Harmful Effects. Natural News. *http://www.naturalnews.com/022630.html.* Accessed July 2010.

2. Lam, M. Estrogen Dominance. Biomedical Labs. 2010. *http://www.biomediclabs.com/estrogen_dominance.* Accessed July 2010.

3. Hull, J. Aspartame – Other Sweeteners. Sweet Poison. 2002. *http://www.sweetpoison.com/aspartame-sweeteners.html* Accessed June 2010.

4. Mercola. Aspartame is, by far, the most dangerous substance on the market that is added to foods. Mercola. 2011. *http://aspartame.mercola.com/* Accessed November 17, 2011.

5. Lorenzo N, Chawla J, et al. Neurologic Effects of Caffeine. Medscape. Nov 2008. *http://emedicine.medscape.com/article/1182710-overview* Accessed June 2010.

6. Suleman A, Siddiqui N. Hemodynamic And Cardiovascular Effects Of Caffeine. Priory. 1995. *http://priory.com/pharmol/caffeine.htm* Accessed June 2010.

7. CocoPure website. *http://www.newvitality.com/shop/coco-pure.aspx* Accessed May 2010.

8. Mercola. Fructose Affects Your Brain Very Differently than Glucose. Mercola. 2011. http://articles.mercola.com/sites/articles/archive/2011/02/28/new-study-*confirms-fructose-affects-your-brain-very-differently-than-glucose.aspx* Accessed November 15, 2011.

9. Murray RK, Bender DA, Botham, KM, et al. Harper's Illustrated Biochemistry. 28th ed. Columbus, OH: Tim MicGraw-Hill: 2009. *http://ksemdoc.files.wordpress.com/2010/02/fructose-metabolism.gif.* Accessed November 15, 2011.

10. Goldberg AL, Etlinger JD, Goldspink DF, et al. Mechanism of work-induced hypertrophy of skeletal muscle [abstract]. Med Sci Sports. 1975; 7(3): 185-98. *http://www.ncbi.nlm.nih.gov/pubmed/128681.* Accessed November 16, 2011.

11. Trudo, M. Self-Myofascial Release. X Factor Fitness Solutions. 2010. *http://www.xfactorfitnesssolutions.com/blog/myofascial-release.* Accessed November 17, 2011.

12. Hernandez JR, Kravitz L. The Mystery of Skeletal Muscle Hypertrophy. University of New Mexico. 2006. Accessed November 17, 2011. *http://www.unm.edu/~lkravitz/Article%20folder/hypertrophy.html.*

13. D'ambrosio F. Posture is Important. Southern California Orthopedic Institute. *http://www.scoi.com/posture.htm* Accessed November 17, 2011.

14. Hirth CJ. Clinical Movement Analysis to Identify Muscle Imbalances and Guide Exercise. NASM. 2007. *http://www.nasm.org/uploadedFiles/NASMORG/objects/downloads/NASM_Clinical_Movement_Analysis%20(PDF,%20411K).pdf.* Accessed November 17, 2011.

15. Exercise Rx. *http://www.exrx.net/ExInfo/Posture.html* Accessed November 2011.

I CAN DO ALL THINGS THROUGH CHRIST WHO STRENGTHENS ME. PHILIPPIANS 4:13

Many Thanks to

First, Foremost and most important, My Lord as Savior, Jesus Christ. Because of him, I can do all things!

My parents Barb and Bill Clark for believing in me and supporting me in all my dreams

Roger Semsch, Powerhouse Gym. You have given me a platform to change lives and live out the path I know God has placed me on. Your assistance with my nutrition and your teaching has helped to make me what I am today.

Amy Lescher, you are a beautiful champion and I was blessed to have your help with the book.

Libby Herman for your diligence, hard work and dedication to helping me live my dreams and change the lives of all those I work with. Your research is helping all of us live healthier lives.

Brendan O'Neil with Kor Integrated Fitness for helping me to see that training has many paths, but without proper flexibility, alignment and posture you have nothing.

My staff of trainers. You inspire me to be better. You bless me daily watching lives change in your hands. God has given each of us exactly what we need to get each new person exactly where they need to go!

Thank you Matt Martin for taking my business to the next level and positioning us to be able to change more lives than ever before. You are such a blessed addition to my team.

Thanks Jeff for all that you have done to help with this. Without you I wouldn't have this book.

Practitioners

Dr. Anna Bone D.O.
Bone Chiropractic
7734 Watson Road
St. Louis, MO 63119
314-961-1807

Dr. Christian Wessling M.D.
7979 Big Bend Boulevard
Webster Groves, MO 63119
314-961-6631

Dr. Maureen Stoffa M.D.
3009 N.Ballas Road Suite 100B
St. Louis, MO 63131
314-432-1111

Dr. Richard Bligh M.D. MBA
777 S. New Ballas Road
Suite 200E
Town and Country, MO 63141
314-994-1536

Sayers Brook Bison Ranch
Grass Fed Bison shipped to your door
573-438-4449
Sayersbrook.com

Marty Henderson Photography
314-249-5509
All Fitness and headshot pictures taken by Marty

Heaven Sent Photography
by Meredith Struebing
636-255-4679
hsphoto@charter.net
All kitchen and grocery photos taken by Meredith

Healing Touch Limited
Massage Therapy
David Meyerkord
314-781-8337

Eric Freukes L.M.M.T.
Licensed Medical Massage Therapist
27 years experience
314-651-8151
eric@ericfreukes.com

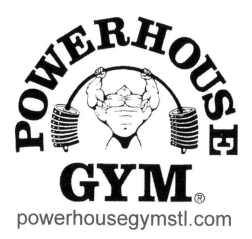

powerhousegymstl.com

Debbie Portell

PERSONAL TRAINING & NUTRITION

debbiecooperportell@yahoo.com

(636) 299-2208

www.debbieportell.com

Phillipians 4:13

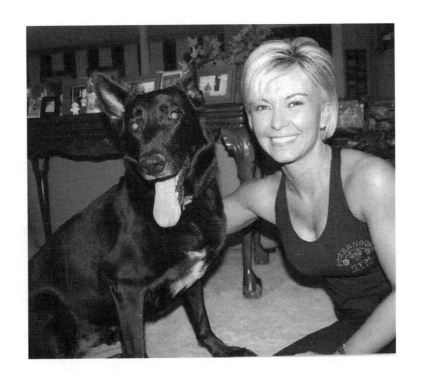

"I can do all things through Christ who strengthens me."

-Philippians 4:13